The
HOSPICE
CHOICE

In Pursuit of a Peaceful Death

Marcia Lattanzi-Licht

with

John J. Mahoney and

Galen W. Miller

A Fireside Book
Published by Simon & Schuster

FIRESIDE
Rockefeller Center
1230 Avenue of the Americas
New York, NY 10020

Manufactured in the United States of America
3   5   7   9   10   8   6   4

Library of Congress Cataloging-in-Publication Data
Lattanzi-Licht, Marcia E.
The hospice choice : in pursuit of a peaceful death / Marcia Lattanzi-Licht,
John J. Mahoney, Galen W. Miller.
p. cm.
Includes bibliographical references and index.
1. Hospice care. I. Mahoney, John J., date. II. Miller, Galen W.
(Galen Willis). III. Title.
R726.8.L37 1997   362.1'756—dc21
97-36948 CIP
ISBN 0-684-82269-5

Every effort has been made to contact copyright holders; in the event of an
inadvertent omission or error, please notify the publisher. The author is
grateful for permission to use excerpts from the following works:

Quoted from Rabbi Tsvi Blanchard's address given at Stern College for
Women of Yeshiva University, April 24, 1994, and reprinted with permission by Simon & Schuster from *Because God Loves Stories: An Anthology of*

(continues on page 280)

To our loving families

The History of the National Hospice Organization Logo

The logo was designed for NHO and donated in 1977 by S. Neil Fujita, an artist with Ruder & Finn, Inc., an international public relations firm. In September 1981, the NHO logo was officially registered as the property of the National Hospice Organization.

Chosen from several designs presented by Mr. Fujita, the logo seemed to best symbolize what the hospice concept represents. The NHO logo is meant to have a universal interpretation. The following interpretation of the design was presented at a hospice conference in Connecticut in November 1977 by Dr. Mary Cummings:

> The themes of hospice are repeated in different ways in the logo. The white in the center is a shining light representing hope, life, and love:
>
> - Hope, in relief of symptoms
> - Life, not in extension, but in enhancement
> - Love within patients, families, and providers
>
> The circle is a continuum of life and whatever comes after. The petals represent the physical, psychological, social, and spiritual components of hospice given to each hospice patient and family. The logo as a whole embodies the philosophy of hospice.

CONTENTS

INTRODUCTION

So there are stories that tell about holding people while they cry with the pains of this world, and then there are other stories that show the possibility of really coming full circle, of being transformed. The stories show us what it means to actually be able to touch all parts of ourselves and bring them together, and to access what is available not just in our own memory, but all across the spectrum of our family's memory, of our community's memory, of the human race's memory, and perhaps in spiritual domains we can only begin to understand.

—RABBI TSVI BLANCHARD

IT IS NEVER easy to enter the world of someone who is dying. And that is precisely what hospice care is about: entering the home and lives of a family where a loved one is living out the last portion of life. The end of life is a highly personal and intimate time. The experience of caring for a loved one who is dying is only spoken of in short, sweeping ways to the larger circle of people we know, or in quiet, honest, searching talks with those few close people who ask and are willing to listen. *The Hospice Choice: In Pursuit of a Peaceful Death* invites you into the experiences of families facing the death of a loved one.

The dying process pushes us to the edges of our understandings and leaves us standing there feeling alone and lost. There is a longing for closeness and a need to bridge the separations, to try to express all that has been unspoken, or to repeat the important things for emphasis. During the time my precious friend Barbara Carnahan was dying and a hospice patient, she made valiant efforts to communicate to the people she loved. Intentionally, she told the people she loved about the things she appreciated and valued in her relationships with us. There were intimate conversations, phone calls, and loving, painstakingly written notes.

Barbara was diagnosed and died with hospice support during the writing of this book. An adaptation of her story is told in one of the chapters. And yet, telling the story of Barbara's hospice experience shows you only a vignette of her life. It's not possible to represent the unrepeatable qualities and contributions that are now her legacy or to truly show what it was like to watch her face her illness and her dying.

When I think about the time that Barbara was dying, I remember the sense of unreality surrounding her illness. It was like being part of a television drama that we would never have chosen to watch. How could the friend who used her strength as a massage therapist to bring healing to others be so ill herself? How could her sparkling energy, like the bright purple, red, and turquoise colors she always wore, be fading? Barbara was my very close friend for the better part of two decades and I counted on her in good and difficult times. We looked forward to growing old together, and I still have an image in my mind of us sitting on the deck together, colored by advancing years, smiling and telling stories.

I met Barbara through our hospice work, and I remember our shared dedication and seriousness. There were long walks in our neighborhood with talk about our triumphs and struggles. (The struggles often involved men.) There were hikes, bike rides, cross-country skiing, movies, holiday meals, birthday celebrations, country-western dancing, book swapping, telephone calls, long talks, and everyday stories. It's the stories that I treasure the most. And the images that are part of the stories stay with me, floating through my days on the breezes of memory and time.

Barbara and I raised children who were close in age, and we commiserated when they were adolescents and rejoiced as they grew. I remember her being at my home the morning after my seventeen-year-old daughter, Ellen, was killed by a drunk driver. And all the other days after that. Her friendship was solid ground, where I could stand in a time when very little felt certain.

As the years passed, she delighted in my marriage and our circle of kinship grew wider. There are always surprises involved in a deep friendship, and the wondrous realizations that you can truly count on your friend's help. When I brought my husband, Mike, home after his cancer surgery, Barbara had a meal waiting in the refrigerator. And she came by every week after his treatments and visited briefly with us, bringing flowers or treats. Barbara was a truly gracious, generous soul and a consummate giver of gifts. I feel about Barbara in a similar way to how I see my daughter Ellen's absence. I miss their loving presences in my life, and I know that missing them will continue to be a part of my life. Barbara, like Ellen, was a great gift to my life.

While Barbara's crippling illness limited her, she learned to express and expand her humor and her awareness. She lived her final months gracefully, and with a full heart—the way she had lived her life. I remember wanting to tell some of the hospice professionals about what an unusual and remarkable woman Barbara was. I didn't need to do that. In spite of her physical and functional diminishment, Barbara's essence was apparent. Her being nourished people during her living and her dying, and her memory continues to do so.

Another dear friend, Al Lane, died with hospice support during the writing of this book. Al and Betty, his wife of fifty-four years, lived the last months of his life together, enjoying as many moments as possible, wishing they could have had more time. The death of these two friends sharpened my understanding of hospice in a very personal way. There were many powerful reminders in my involvement with both Barbara's and Al's last months. Hospice made a great difference for both of them and made it easier for their loved ones. I was reminded of how well the approach to care that hospice involves actually works, and of its practical and symbolic value for families.

Understanding hospice involves understanding people who are in the middle of experiencing that unimaginable time surrounding death. Stories offer a personal lens for looking into the experience of dying and losing a loved one from several perspectives, especially those of family members. Carl Jung believed that what is most personal is also highly universal. *The Hospice Choice: In Pursuit of a Peaceful Death* depicts the hospice experience through the stories of families who have received hospice care. There are also stories told from the vantage point of hospice volunteers and another from that of a hospice nurse.

One of the modern pioneering voices who encouraged the understanding of death's importance in our lives, Herman Feifel, observed that "people die in notably personal ways." These stories are a collage of different experiences and people, based upon years of professional and personal work with dying and grief. While there are commonalities, there are also unique and unrepeating aspects of each story.

Death and grief create moving and deep human dramas. Families invite hospice into their distinctive dramas, allowing hospice professionals and volunteers to be present for the all-important climax and ending of a person's life. In any drama, the climax, that part we remember most, is when the potent themes emerge and stand in bold relief. In a *Casablanca*-like way, we stand to meet head-on the demands of parting, summoning the courage and grace to leave or to watch the person we love depart. These one-and-only moments become key memories that replay often during the early days and months of grief. We carry them with us throughout our remaining lifetimes.

Experiences around death and grief forge the themes that become the guiding images for our lives. Hospice presents families the opportunity to play out their own themes, to sing their own songs. These themes, while deeply personal, resonate with our own experiences. Such pervasive themes as isolation, belonging, impermanence, and individual worth are found in the stories you'll read here. Hopeful themes of powerlessness and choice, searching, reconciliation, and welcoming life also appear in each of the descriptions. The central motif woven throughout all these stories echoes the impact and ripple effects of love and loss.

If there is one image of hospice that stays with me, it is the image of a competent stranger coming to the door, saying, "I'm here to help." The relief and power which that statement affords the family is difficult to measure. Hospice care offers families the comfort of feeling less alone.

The compassionate care that hospice represents is not easily defined or provided. By its very nature, care that is compassionate must be shaped to fit the individual needs and values of the people and families involved. Perhaps that is the most significant element of hospice care. Instead of asking the dying person and family members to fit into a caregiving system, hospice care extends services around their unique situation and values. So, the man dying of lung cancer may choose to continue to smoke up until the time of his death, or the woman dying from metastatic breast cancer may choose to continue taking her alternative treatments. Hospice professionals and volunteers focus on the individual and family's world, encouraging personal choices and meaningful experiences around the process of dying. In the presence of hospice's quiet yet strong support, families have the chance to be together in exceptional ways in the time still available to them. The hospice choice may be one of the most human and loving possibilities available at the end of life's journey.

—MARCIA LATTANZI-LICHT

We have a long way to go. So let us hasten along the road, the road of human tenderness and generosity. Groping, we may find one another's hands in the dark.

—EMILY GREEN BALCH,
1946 Nobel Peace Laureate

ACKNOWLEDGMENTS

BECAUSE THE PRINCIPLE of teamwork is central to hospice care, it was a living reality for the development and writing of this book. When Simon & Schuster contacted the National Hospice Organization regarding their interest in a book on hospice care for consumers, Galen Miller was the project visionary and enthusiastically guided its development. Jay Mahoney brought his focused, grounding style to the book, and his encouragement helped move the project to reality.

Galen was supported by Bob Ward, not only in his patience and understanding, but in his willingness to read and comment on the evolving chapters.

Jay Mahoney relied on the generous and sustaining assistance that Laura Mahoney gave so capably, adding the perspective of her own hospice experience.

This book benefited from the generous help of the staff of the National Hospice Organization. Special thanks to Cathy Anouar, who expertly and cheerfully engineered the editing and final production of the manuscript. Jan Goudreau, librarian for the National Hospice Organization, worked to get permissions for the many quotes used in the book. Many thanks to Debb Stipp, David Schneider, Susan Buckley, Samira Beckwith, Sarah Hill, and the NHO staff and board of directors for their encouragement. Caroline Sutton, our editor at Simon & Schuster, gave us sound support during the writing and her skillful editing suggestions helped fashion a stronger book.

Ramona Miller and Julia Dickens read the entire manuscript and offered helpful consumer perspectives.

Many of the people who reviewed the stories in this book have been part of my extended family and circle of friends for many years. They are precious friends and colleagues who gave ongoing support for this book. I met most of them during the years of my involvement with hospice. Anne Compton, Connie Studer, and Diane Coffelt offered valuable insight and gave excellent critical feedback on the manuscript. Mary Hale, Bernice Catherine Harper, Donna and Charles Corr, Marie Gates, and Ann Luke offered their guidance and experienced view on selected chapters. Thora Chinnery, Elizabeth Lane, Elizabeth Licht, and Eva Steinhardt helped with their reflections on individual chapters. Al Lane, our dear friend of many years, also died during the writing of this book and benefited from hospice services.

The remarkable women of Spirit Walkers: Trudy Hughes, Marlene Wilson, Elsie Richardson, and Barbara Pellochoud were stalwarts of understanding and reassurance, in addition to offering their insights. My dear friend Barbara Carnahan, who I met through hospice work, died as this book was being written. Her journey reconfirmed for me the value of hospice services. Her excitement over my work, even in her final days, was constant. All these people offered their sustaining friendship and unwavering support.

Peggy Richardson, Kim Mooney, and Pat Mehnert, who continue the important work at Hospice of Boulder County, read chapters and gave practical feedback and helpful comments. Lorraine Janis Ellis, Jo Spees, Dale Larson, Steve Connor, Valerie MacLaren, and Karen Spehr, friends and colleagues of many years, offered ongoing enthusiasm and encouragement for my work.

It was possible for me to write stories about families because I have had such rich experiences in my own family of origin, in the family that included my two children, and in the larger family that involves a community of friends who have stood with me during these more than twenty years of my involvement with hospice care. My parents, Chester and Helen Jaworski, and my sisters Lori Monthei and Christine

Rejniak have been constant in their love and always encourage my best efforts. Lori's friendship has been an ongoing foundation of my life.

Most of all, a heart full of thanks to my husband, Mike Licht, who was my faithful editor and wise companion throughout the writing of this book. Even when writing intruded upon the quality of our day-to-day life, Mike was at my side every step of the way. His strong love and helpfulness sustain me. He is at the heart of all that I do.

Steve Lattanzi, my son, journeyed with me through this hospice project, as well as the years of my involvement with hospice. His appreciation of my work, and his love and belief in me throughout my career, have made a tremendous difference.

My daughter, Ellen Lattanzi, taught me a great deal about life and love in the seventeen years she was with us. Her life was a gift and her death has had an immeasurable influence upon my being, including the way I see death, grief, and the world of hospice care. Most of what I know I learned with or from my children.

What Galen, Jay, and I have written in this book is what we know about hospice and the impact of dying and grief. My heartfelt gratitude to Jay and Galen for the opportunity to work with them, and to all the people who encircled me with love and patience during the writing of this book. This book is a testimony to all the dying and grieving people I have been privileged to walk with during the years. I will always be grateful to all the people who invited me into the personal world of their sorrow and searching. I remember their stories. This book witnesses their love and honors their courage.

—MARCIA LATTANZI-LICHT

Chapter One

SAYING GOOD-BYE TO DAD:
A Family Journeys Together

Everything is changing for Garfield Platt and his family. Just two weeks before he was diagnosed with inoperable lung cancer, Garfield Platt was out in deep snow saving the newborn calves on his small cattle ranch. Now, five months later, at 71, his life is slipping away as quickly as the morning mist on the prairie he has always called home.

Proud of his hard work and modest successes, Garfield Platt is dedicated to his ranch and his family. His wife, Norma, has been with him for forty-seven years, and their relationship reflects their quiet, steady natures. Norma and Garfield have two grown children, Melanie and Bob. Busy with demands of their careers and families, both Melanie and Bob keep in close contact with their parents but are less close to each other.

Melanie, the oldest, lives 700 miles away and visits two or three times a year. A corporate attorney, she is divorced and has no children. Bob, his parent's favorite as a child, is a program manager for a large computer manufacturer. He lives sixty miles away with his wife and 10-year-old son. Since his father has become more ill, Bob visits at least once a week. Garfield would like Bob to visit more frequently and stay longer, and often chides him about being in such a hurry.

In spite of the radiation treatments, Garfield's breathing is becoming more and more difficult. For the past ten weeks, he has needed constant oxygen and he finds wheeling around the tank bothersome. His weight is dropping rapidly and he's increasingly tired and depleted. An independent rancher who could handle the crises of severe winter storms and drought, Garfield feels his life is out of control.

At Garfield's visit to the oncologist, Dr. Miller recommended the care of the local hospice. While Garfield did not fully understand the services, he trusts Dr. Miller. And, Norma is needing more help and time to do errands. One of the ways that Norma copes with the pressures of ranch life is by visiting with the local store merchants and neighbors that she would see while shopping.

When the hospice nurse and social worker come by for the initial visit, both Norma and Garfield are apprehensive. They listen as the nurse and social worker describe the home-care services and the support that hospice offers. Norma is openly relieved and eager for some help. Garfield has numerous questions and is concerned about the people who will be coming into their home. While they are friendly with neighbors, the Platts are private and independent people who do little formal socializing.

As the hospice nurse, Doris, examines Garfield physically, she soon discovers through careful assessment that he is experiencing a fairly constant low-level pain. Garfield describes his pain to the nurse as a gnawing pressure in his lungs and ranks it as a three or four on a ten-point scale that ranges from a mild headache (one) to unbearable pain (ten). They also discuss his shortness of breath, which is creating restlessness and difficulty sleeping.

The hospice nurse continues to ask Mr. Platt about his other concerns. Reluctantly, he admits that he is also having difficulty with constipation, and that he does not enjoy eating much because it seems like too much effort lately. When they talk about the seriousness of his illness, Mr. Platt speaks about licking the cancer. He then concedes that he is very tired. "Sometimes it's hard to go on. One of the things I know from ranching is how to deal with difficult times, but this has thrown me for a loop. I just don't know what to do."

At the same time, out in the living room, Susan, the hospice social worker, asks Norma about how she is handling the physical demands of Garfield's illness, and what types of support she would find helpful. Norma says that she is feeling overwhelmed by Garfield's weakness and irritability, and tearfully admits that sometimes it is hard not to snap back at him. The social worker agrees that full-time caregiving creates a level of distress that most people find difficult to tolerate without an occasional break. She offers the availability of a hospice volunteer to come by once or twice a week. Norma thinks it would be good for Garfield to have someone to talk to or play cards with while she does her errands.

Norma and Garfield are members of the local Methodist church. They had attended regularly in the past, but have not been to church for the past four months. Inquiring about support from the church, the social worker learns that their pastor knows of Garfield's illness, but not of his decline. Norma hopes that he will come out for a visit to their home and agrees to have the hospice chaplain contact their pastor and arrange for him to visit.

The nurse and social worker explain the services to the family, and give them a written pamphlet outlining the Medicare Hospice Benefit. Garfield questions the costs of hospice and Norma is interested to know what nursing services will be available. Even though Garfield is still mobile, he only leaves home for his appointments with the oncologist. "I've always been a man who loved his home, and this is the only place where I want to be now."

After a brief planning discussion, the family and the hospice professionals decide upon twice-weekly nursing visits at the outset. The volunteer will visit once or twice a week, and the social worker will be involved if needed.

Within the first seventy-two hours of hospice's involvement, Garfield begins taking regular doses of an oral narcotic analgesic that Dr. Miller has prescribed. It is adjusted to his specific needs and soon controls his pain. When Garfield initially expressed concern about the addictive nature of the medication, Doris, the hospice nurse, explained that morphine has few side effects and would allow Garfield to stay awake and alert. She went over the possible side effects, and pointed out that it was most important for Garfield to feel comfortable.

Norma is able to help Garfield with his shower for the first two weeks of hospice care. After that, a nursing assistant, Cathy, is assigned to assist Garfield three times a week with personal care.

The hospice volunteer, Dave, comes by once or twice a week for a couple of hours to play rummy or blackjack with Garfield for as long as his energy holds up. Dave teases Garfield about quitting when Dave is winning, so they are keeping a running score of the game. Usually, after a half hour, they sit together and listen to a local radio station, commenting to each other on items of interest. Three weeks later, Garfield is too weak to play cards, and finds it hard to engage in even small bits of conversation. Short of breath even with increased oxygen, Garfield tells Dave, "I feel like I can't say too much anymore. I do like to have you here, though." Dave continues to visit and reads the local paper to Garfield, or watches television with him.

The following week, Melanie comes out for a three-day weekend visit and attends to her parent's legal affairs and will. During the visit, Melanie and Bob have harsh words with each other about their relationships with their parents. Long-standing resentments boil over, and afterward, Bob and Melanie are not speaking to each other.

Both parents are distressed over the conflict, but feel powerless to know how to make things better. After the second day of Melanie's stay, Mr. Platt speaks openly to the hospice nurse during her regular visit. "Things are just too complicated, and this is too hard on Norma and the family." Listening, the nurse reassures Garfield that his family will work things out, with the hospice team available to help make things smoother.

The hospice nurse remarks to Melanie that the stresses of seeing her father so ill may be greater than she realizes. She suggests that since Melanie will be in town for one more day that she and Bob meet with the hospice social worker to discuss family decisions, their father's care, and any other concerns or questions. Reluctantly, Melanie and Bob agree, and Susan, the hospice social worker, spends time with them clarifying their concerns for their father and their roles in helping the family navigate this difficult time. Both acknowledge that they feel helpless and are struggling to deal with the loss of their favorite parent. "There's no one like Dad," Melanie tells Susan. "He always seemed so strong and invincible, and he made everything right for us when we were upset or discouraged. It's hard to imagine this family without him. He's the glue that holds us together."

Recognizing the extra burden of responsibility that Bob must feel, Melanie thanks him for being available to their parents. While there is still tension, some of the overt conflicts are eased. Melanie promises to come back at whatever point Bob feels she would be needed, asking that he give her a couple of days notice if possible. Knowing he has some backup with their parents is the most important thing for Bob because he does not want to be criticized or blamed for decisions after the fact. Bob and Melanie decide to speak on the phone every other day to keep up with the changes.

When Bob visits his parents every weekend, he feels a sense of shock at his father's physical condition and diminished appearance. Garfield looks weaker, even though he is still four inches taller and outweighs Bob. Spending his time checking on the maintenance of the ranch and other tangible business needs his mother has, Bob usually avoids significant contact with his father. He lingers in the kitchen, typically avoiding the bedroom where his father spends his time watching television or dozing on and off. Each visit, Bob goes back for a couple of brief exchanges with his dad.

This Friday, Cathy, the hospice nursing assistant, comes into the kitchen after she has finished Garfield's bath and asks Bob if he would like to shave his father. Looking as if he is too embarrassed to say no, Bob reluctantly walks back to the bedroom where his father is resting. It takes only a few minutes with his hands applying shaving cream and stroking the razor across Garfield's withered face for Bob to realize that his father is still here, still the man he knows. They talk about the ranch and retell the stories that are a family's richest inheritance. Bob jokes with his father about whether this shave would meet the strict standards Garfield had always set for the chores on the ranch. When they are finished, Garfield asks Bob to take him in the wheelchair to the living room so that he can look out on his herd and the fields.

As they sit near the window in silence, Garfield looks over at his son and tells him that although he had wished Bob would have taken over the ranch, Garfield is proud of the man Bob is, and of his successes. Then Garfield asks Bob to take care of his mother, to make sure that she will be all right. Looking straight at his father, Bob promises "You can count on me, Dad." Those few moments hold a lifetime's worth of importance to Bob, who could now be the strong one, the one to help his dad.

Bob asks Garfield about being in the living room, and he admits that he enjoys looking out on the fields he had walked and worked for more than fifty years. "I've always loved to watch the sun draw shadows on the grasses. There's magic in the way light changes the face of the prairie," Garfield tells his son. Bob promises to call hospice and ask for a hospital bed to be delivered, and to have it put by the living room window.

Bob feels different as he drives home, as if he had visited an emotional place he hadn't known before today. He can't picture life without his father. It will be hard to explain to his wife, Nancy, and his son, Paul, what this visit has meant. How could they prepare for the days ahead, for Garfield's death?

Paul had always been fascinated by his grandfather's stories and looked forward to working alongside him every summer. There would be no summers like that again.

Melanie is in a gray space that holds flashes of images of her gravely ill father and the finality that she can't yet absorb. At work, the demands of her job take her away from the consuming thoughts that are edged with fear. There is a pressured feeling that pulls Melanie forward through her days.

Susan had given Melanie the phone number of a local hospice that offers a family member's group. The next week, Melanie called Bob to say that she had attended a session at the hospice near her office. Melanie found it both striking and reassuring to be in a room where so many family members were dealing with the same problems. Now, she is so busy at work that she doesn't know if she will have the time to go again.

Melanie phones her mother or brother every day. This week, Bob tells Melanie that he has had angry words with their mother twice recently. After a meeting with the hospice nurse, they agreed to have a respite nurse help for two or three nights a week. Bob feels worried about their mother, seeing how tired and how much older she looks. He also tells Melanie that their father is growing weaker and nearer to the end of his life.

As Garfield's life slowly ebbs, he is comfortable and sleeps more. The last two weeks he spends most of his days in the recliner, or in bed, propped up by pillows almost in a sitting position. Garfield seems calm and uses his limited breath and energy to speak with those he loves. When their pastor visits again, Garfield tells him that he is trying to stay alive until his forty-eighth wedding anniversary the next week. The minister reassures Garfield that his intentions matter and they pray together in silence.

When Bob is at the ranch the following Saturday, Garfield asks him to buy a heart-shaped gold brooch for Norma's anniversary gift. "I want her to have a sign of how much I love her. And see to it that we have things in order to celebrate. Could Nancy handle the meal, and a cake? It means a lot to me to do this for Norma."

"I'll take care of it, Dad. Celebrating together has always been important to our family. We'll make both you and Mom feel special on your day."

As the anniversary draws nearer, Garfield's determination grows. He knows that these months have been rough on Norma. He believes that celebrating their anniversary is one gift he can still give her.

Melanie flies in on Friday for the weekend. The whole family has been making plans to be together on Saturday for the anniversary. They set up the table and eat dinner together in the living room with Garfield. Afterward, Norma unwraps Garfield's present to her, the heart brooch, and reads the card he wrote. Norma tearfully hugs Garfield as he tells her "You will always be my love. I wouldn't have missed the chance to celebrate this anniversary with you for anything."

The following Thursday morning the hospice nurse spends time talking to Norma and tells her that Garfield will probably be with them for just a few more days. The nurse describes the changes that Norma can expect to see in Garfield as his death comes closer. Norma says that she can handle things. Reassuring her that hospice will be available to help, the nurse reminds Norma to call at whatever point she needs someone. While the nurse is still checking on Garfield, Norma calls Bob and asks him to come over after work.

When Garfield dies on Friday evening, both Norma and Bob are with him, sitting next to his bed in the living room. Norma keeps stroking his head and talking to him. His breathing gets rougher and slower, then finally stops. They had called the hospice nurse who is also there with them. Twenty minutes later, Nancy arrives with Melanie from the airport, and the family sits with Garfield's body for a while before they call the funeral director.

The saddened family members, aware of the magnitude of their loss, react with gentleness and love for each other.

There are differences in what each family member wants for the service, but they manage to work together with the funeral director and pastor so that all their wishes are included. Norma wants a cousin to sing a solo and Melanie would like a friend to play a piano piece. Bob and Paul will stain the casket, and put the brand of the family ranch on it. There is a close, tender feeling in the house as neighbors stop by.

Norma is touched by the large turnout for Garfield's funeral, with scores of neighbors and members of the church as well as the hospice nurse and volunteer attending. After the burial and the lunch at the church, the immediate family gathers at the ranch. They discuss plans for the ranch. Since Garfield's illness, a local young man has been successfully managing the ranch, and they decide to ask him to continue on for at least another year. No one wants to give up the family home.

Norma gives her children and grandson each a personal memento of Garfield's. She also asks them if they want any special pieces of his clothing. Norma keeps his favorite flannel shirt and his red wool jacket; the rest of the clothes will eventually be donated to charity.

After everyone goes back home that week, Norma has a difficult time adjusting to the emptiness of her days. It is hard to stop thinking about all that has happened since Garfield became ill less than seven months ago.

The following week another hospice volunteer, Donna, calls and asks to visit Norma. During the visit, she talks with Norma about how she is coping and brings along some written information about the ways people respond to grief. She tells Norma about the various support groups that hospice offers. The hospice social worker had mentioned the groups for widows when she'd called Norma the previous week. Before Donna leaves, Bob phones and Norma tells him that the hospice volunteer is visiting. "I'm so relieved to know that some of the things I've been worried about, like feeling restless, having difficulty concentrating, and waking up during the night are all part of what grieving people experience."

Two months after Garfield's death, Norma attends a bereavement meeting at the hospice office. The speaker focuses on the questions of faith that illness and death bring. Afterward, Norma talks with two widows whom she had known casually at church. The three of them set up a time to go out to dinner together the following week.

Next month Norma is planning to stay with Melanie for a week. She has been encouraging her to visit, and Norma thinks it may help the loneliness. Bob, Nancy, and Paul come by for dinner on Sundays. They are all talking more openly since Garfield's death. Bob says that the one good thing that has come from Garfield's death is that the family has grown closer.

We are all of us calling and calling across the incalculable gulfs which separate us.

—DAVID GRAYSON

A Family Matter

Illness and death affect families, not only individuals. In a time when families are often geographically separate, they are also called upon to be the caregivers for their ill or dying members. Smaller families are also the trend, with fewer hands to do the tasks, fewer people to assume needed roles.

There are some central assumptions or defining elements that we attribute to our involvement in a family. We look for both the basic and strengthening aspects of family:

- A sense of safety
- Belonging
- Acceptance
- Shared responsibilities
- Protection

- Support
- A common history
- Division of roles
- Relationships where we are known, or understood

While most families have significant capacities as well as limitations, it is common to think of one's family in the way that Robert Frost spoke of it in his poem "The Death of the Hired Man": *Home is the place where, when you have to go there, / They have to take you in.*

For many of us, our family is the group that is most available and most reliable in a difficult time. The hospice definition of family includes all those in loving relationships with the person who is dying, the people who can be counted on for caring and support, regardless of blood or legal ties.

In a study of the measures of support, it was found that families were the ones we most frequently turned to in times of need. The things that family members offered that were noted as most helpful were encouragement, emotional support, companionship, help with problem-solving, and tangible aid.[1] Our earliest ancestors banded together in groups to offer each other protection from predators. Perhaps caring for a seriously ill family member is our modern day parallel of gathering together in the presence of a major threat to seek protection, safety, and comfort.

Families at Their Best

Families are the best models of small communities that we have in our current culture. There is shared concern, commitment, and interdependence. Even in families where there have been conflicted or difficult relationships, the constructive elements can still be present, and actually serve as powerful motivators for providing care to an ill or dying family member.

Families and their individual members can be at their best as they face the imminent death of their loved one. Old grievances can be forgotten and inadequacies in the relationship forgiven. In facing the irrevocable loss of a family member, it is possible to put the person's worth and the relationship into a different context. It is also possible for family members to be more generous and open with other members of the family who are not ill.

Families and Time

When we witness a life-threatening illness that diminishes a family member, we often wake up to the fact that the clock is ticking, that our opportunities with the person we love are dwindling. Lacking time or a future, we are more willing to enter into the present and make those moments as good as they can be. The illness and death of a loved one is a one-and-only moment, an unrepeatable time. If we do not participate in that time, there will be no other opportunities with that person.

Families and Caregiving

The delivery of family-centered care, rather than care that focuses solely on the ill person, is a major distinction of hospice. Family members who care for their loved one face a strenuous and stressful experience. The counterbalance to the tremendous effort of caregiving lies in the opportunity to redeem past inadequacies in the relationship with moments of closeness at the end of a loved one's life. Caring for a loved one who is dying diminishes guilt and self-criticism in the time of bereavement.[2] This understanding became an important foundation for the hospice approach.

The momentous nature of the dying process offers opportunities to be with people—opportunities that are unusual in today's world. Most families relate to the dying process as both a difficult and a valuable time. The demands of caregiving can create resentments and anger that compound relationship difficulties. In the final analysis, though, the vast majority of family members who care for a loved one describe high feelings of self-satisfaction and little regret.

That is not to say that family members do not pay a high price in caring for their loved one. They do. The physical demands and the toll of watching someone you love become diminished and unable to function are extraordinary. Family members experience physical stresses and exhaustion, isolation, and spiritual doubts, and must struggle to maintain the quality of their own lives. The caregiving act means, for many, the loss of other parts of their lives. There is no time for everyday activities, and less energy for attention to other family members. While family members have some unique concerns, in many ways they mirror the needs of the person who is dying.

Difficult Family Experiences

A parallel of how families relate to the caregiving experience may be seen in the ways families respond to pregnancy and the birth of a child. Pregnancy and childbirth can be physically difficult and demanding, a time when some daily patterns are altered and life as we knew it changes. There are also positive aspects of the process, and in the aftermath of the labor and birth, mothers and fathers do not forget the discomfort of the experience and the sacrifices involved; rather, they choose to remember the rewards of their efforts.

In the same way, family members do not forget the difficulties involved in caring for a loved one who is dying, and all the many losses and trials along the way. Instead, they can focus on the gratification, comfort, and confidence that can come from having done all they could to care for and be with their loved one until the very end.

Journeying Together

Human beings can be at their best when they are behaving with altruism and commitment to a person they love. Caring for a loved one who is dying reflects the highest commitment we can make to each other as human beings. People who are dying fear being alone or abandoned. The metaphor embodied in the concept of hospice is that of a journey. Inherent in the caregiving process is the message *"I will journey with you."* This reassurance is what we all hope for, and what is difficult to ask for without feeling like a burden to loved ones.

One of the major difficulties that dying people negotiate is the experience of being the recipient of the care and concern—and sometimes even the sympathy—of others. By receiving the care of others, the person who is ill gives an important gift. Viktor Frankl, a noted psychiatrist who survived Auschwitz, believed that the person who is ill helps the one who is well find meaning.[3] While there is a great generosity involved in the caregiving effort, there is also immeasurable beneficence in allowing others to care for us. Some spiritual writers see receiving as the highest form of giving. The person who is ill and graciously receives the care of others gives them the gift of feeling good about their actions and contributions.

In reflecting upon the important times of our lives, inevitably people remember the imprint of times surrounding the death of a loved one. Caring for someone you love during their final days is a complex experience filled with frustration as well as potential for satisfaction and meaning. Perhaps the most enduring legacy of caregiving is the meaning that we derive from the experience. Frankl offers three avenues for discovering meaning: *creating a work or doing a deed, experiencing something or encountering someone,* and *the attitude we take toward unavoidable suffering.*[4] Each of these opportunities is available both to family members caring for their loved one and to the person who is dying. When we are asked to do more than we may want or feel able to do, we forge a sense of self that is changed by the intensity and power of the experience.

Changing Ways of Being Together

People who are dying do not have the energy to maintain the typical set of human defenses. There is a scraping away of the layers of protection that we cover ourselves with in ordinary times. Faced with the loss of our health and our daily roles, perhaps we become our most basic selves.

Dame Cicely Saunders, the English physician who was a creator of the modern-day hospice movement, said that hospice workers were "missing their outer layer of skin." The implication of this statement is that hospice work demands openness and involvement with people at times of their lives when they are very vulnerable. Family members, like hospice workers, need to have a considerable degree of personal accessibility and a lack of rigid defenses to be able to effectively enter into these sacred and important times.

While the concerns of family members may seem different from those of the person who is dying, they all center around dealing with losses. As the Platts did, family members must also watch and witness the deterioration of their loved one, a very distressing experience. They must address the spiritual and emotional reactions they will experience as they watch their loved one die. Eventually, they must separate and begin planning for an uncertain future without that special person.

Goals of Hospice Care

Hospices have been at the forefront of efforts to involve and include families in providing care. The partnership formed between a family and hospice professionals and volunteers can insure quality care for a person who is dying. Supportive services are designed to offer information and backup to family members so that they will be more able to care for their loved one. Overall, hospice care focuses on addressing some key goals:

1. To support individuals and families in the process of coping with dying
2. To enhance quality of life through comfort care rather than curative treatment
3. To aggressively treat and expertly manage all pain and physical symptoms associated with an individual's dying
4. To care for the whole person, addressing physical, emotional, psychological, spiritual, and social concerns through an interdisciplinary team approach
5. To sustain the individual's and family members' sense of autonomy, individuality, self-worth, and security
6. To acknowledge and offer support for individuals and their family members facing the losses and grief involved with dying and the death of a loved one
7. To offer bereavement support for family members following the death of their loved one
8. To be a positive influence upon the understanding, compassionate treatment and care of the dying and bereaved

These broad-reaching goals are the foundation for hospice services and activities.

Pain Management

Vigilant attention to physical symptoms is at the core of hospice services. A dying person *can* obtain effective pain relief. Because so many people fear the pain that may surround the process of dying, the comprehensive management of pain and other symptoms offers tangible reassurance and comfort. Pain related to a disease often begins before a person is dying. The person who is ill needs to communicate pain levels to the physician at the point when they begin to interfere with functioning, activities, mood, or quality of daily life. Family members are often the best observers of these changes and can be advocates for their loved one regarding pain management with the physician.

The hospice approach to pain management involves some key elements and understandings:

- Pain management includes facilitating optimal comfort, functional ability, and quality of life
- Thorough and ongoing assessment of the pain, the disease process and medical problems
- Belief in the ill person's report of their pain
- Analgesic drugs are taken around the clock at conveniently scheduled intervals to prevent the recurrence of pain
- Medications and dosages that maintain a desired level of alertness and the ability to engage in waking activities as well as to enjoy a peaceful night's sleep
- Use of convenient, least invasive routes of administration (usually the oral route)
- Recognition of individual differences in the perception and responses to pain and its treatment
- Prevention and management of side effects associated with analgesics
- Providing pain prevention and sustained pain relief
- Integrated approaches to cancer pain, including pharmacological, systemic, and anti-cancer therapies, can be effective in an estimated 85–95 percent of people[5]
- Pain and its treatment interact with other physical symptoms like fatigue, weakness, dyspnea, nausea, constipation, or impaired thinking

Since pain is a highly personal and subjective experience, emotional, social, or spiritual influences are involved. Pain invades a person's world, crowding out possibilities for enjoyment of life. Effective pain management is both a science and an art. It is an intensive effort that involves knowledge, careful assessment, and follow-up along with an understanding of the dying person as a unique individual.

Barriers to Pain Management

Pain is often undertreated because of inadequate knowledge about chronic pain management. Pain is also rarely visible, except in nonverbal expressions, like facial grimacing, which is a classic indicator of pain. Unwarranted fears about side effects or addiction can keep the person who is ill or family members from following through with prescribed dosages and schedules of analgesics. Addiction is not a legitimate concern related to narcotic analgesics since research has shown that it rarely occurs.[6] Tolerance, or decreasing results from a drug across time, can occur. Dependence creates a psychological response to absence of the drug. Dependence implies that the use of a particular medication must be tapered off slowly if it will be discontinued for any reason.

Pain Assessment

One of the major barriers to optimal pain management involves inadequate assessment of the intensity, character, location, and quality of the pain. The hospice nurse asks the dying person about the location, duration, onset, and the severity of the pain. The intensity of a person's pain is typically measured on a numerical scale ranging from zero to ten. A rating of one to four is considered mild pain, five to six is moderate pain, and seven to ten is severe pain. A pain rating of five or more defines substantial pain, or pain that interferes significantly with the person's quality of life. Substantial pain demands attention. All members of the hospice team, including volunteers, are taught to look for the presence of physical pain or other significant physical symptoms in their work with persons who are dying. Pain intensity ratings at various points in the day, related to activities and events, are important.

Pain and Suffering

Looking at the experience of pain in a person who is dying involves seeing him or her in the light of a personal history, family, and cultural beliefs about pain; the social and functional environment; and the meanings that the person attributes to the pain. Pain and suffering are frequently believed to be the same experience. Eric Cassell distinguishes suffering as the distress created by an "actual or perceived threat to the integrity or continued existence of the whole person."[7]

Suffering goes beyond the need for the management of physical pain to the human need for communication, recognition, and compassion surrounding the conflicts, losses, and loneliness involved in the process of dying.

A Plan for Care

The hospice team collaborates on an ongoing basis, and in concert with the family physician, to design an individualized plan of care. Taking into account physical, social, religious and cultural variables and values, the plan of care addresses the unique concerns of the person who is dying as well as those of the family. A plan of care offers a map for both the family receiving services and the hospice team members. Aimed at insuring continuity of care and accountability, the plan of care identifies:

- Needs both of the person who is dying and of the family
- Realistic, achievable goals and objectives
- Agreed-upon outcomes
- Mix and frequency of services and the level of care to be provi ed
- Prescribed medications, treatments, and required medical equipment

- Individual and family understanding, agreement, and involvement with the plan of care.[8]

Hospice Support

Hospice care fits the image of a theater production in which hospice staff and volunteers are the stage crew responsible for props, lighting, cue cards, and all the logistical elements required for the performance. Family members are the actors, writers, and directors, producing their own drama reflecting their history and relationships. In concert with that image, the person who is ill and dying and the family members play the central and determining roles, while the hospice team provides the technical and emotional support to assist that family.

Hospices typically offer families a wide range of supportive efforts that include:

- Information
- Listening
- Guidance
- Specific instruction, teaching
- Respite care
- Stress management
- Modeling of effective caregiving techniques and approaches
- Advocacy
- Feedback
- Encouragement

The family members receive care and support so that they can give the best possible care to the person who is ill. Hospice forms a circle of support around the family as they care for their loved one. In essence, one community supports another community, one network sustains the other.

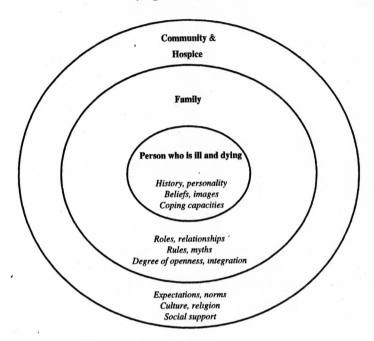

Community &
Hospice

Family

Person who is ill and dying

History, personality
Beliefs, images
Coping capacities

Roles, relationships
Rules, myths
Degree of openness, integration

Expectations, norms
Culture, religion
Social support

The Hospice Circle of Support

Few families and few people have adequate support during the most painful times of their lives. In her troubling novel *Braided Lives*, Marge Piercy reminded us that in difficult times "we need goodwill far more than we have ever earned."

Unique Elements of Hospice

The experience of a major illness means involvement with medical care providers from a variety of backgrounds or specialties. Changes in the delivery of health care have also brought about a shift from inpatient care to outpatient and home-care services. Many home-care programs offer nursing-care support, including nursing assistants, and, occasionally, respite care. Hospice is unique in its commitment to address the broad range of human needs in the challenging terrain of terminal illness and death. Because hospice focuses on *whole person* care, special attention is paid to psychological, emotional, and spiritual needs. *Volunteers,* a distinctive part of the hospice team and the circle of care, work with families both before the death of their loved one and in the time of bereavement. The focus on *family-centered care* led to the development of *bereavement services,* perhaps one of the most differentiating aspects of hospice. A principle of hospice care centers around accessing, involving, and supplementing the family's existing support, not replacing it.

The Contract of Caring

The unspoken contract in close relationships includes being available to each other in times of great need, no matter how difficult or complicated that may be for us. This is a variation of the traditional wedding promise of "till death do us part." We know, whether we acknowledge it or not in our conscious awareness, that in every close relationship one of us will watch the other leave, one of us will say good-bye to another at the time of death.

One of our greatest fears around a terminal illness and the dying process involves feeling alone or abandoned. The metaphor that hospice embodies in the statement "I will journey with you" recognizes the fears of the family members as well, and acknowledges their needs on the journey as the primary caregivers. We cannot take away the illness and the distress that it brings, but we can be with people as they face the difficulties and uncertainties along the way.

> *I gain strength, courage and confidence by every experience in which I must stop and look fear in the face . . . I say to myself, I've lived through this and can take the next thing that comes along . . . We must do the things we think we cannot do.*
>
> —ELEANOR ROOSEVELT

Chapter Two

HOSPICE CARE
An Informed Choice

*Death is a natural part of life, which we all surely have to face
sooner or later. To my mind, there are two ways we can deal
with it while we are alive. We can either choose to ignore it or
we can confront the prospect of our own death and, by thinking
clearly about it, try to minimize the suffering that it can bring.
However, in neither of these ways can we actually overcome it.*

—The 14th Dalai Lama, in the Foreword to
The Tibetan Book of Living and Dying
by Sogyal Rinpoche

THE OBITUARY READ that Donald Morris died in
Parkview Hospital following a lengthy illness. The notice
stated that he was survived by his wife of forty-seven years,
Jean, his sons Michael and Robert, and five grandchildren.
The obituary did not mention that Don died an unnecessarily
typical death.

Don died in the hospital six months after his first admission. He had been admitted to the hospital two other times
during the course of his illness. The second time he was
admitted he spent ten days in an intensive care unit. The last
time he was admitted to the hospital he spent four weeks
there, was resuscitated once, and then slipped into a coma for
a week prior to dying. While in a coma, Don received food
and liquids through a tube. According to his family, Don suf-

fered from moderate to severe pain almost until the day he
died. Was Don's death all too typical? Was all this suffering
necessary? Did Don have other options?

In the last six months of his life, Don spent almost sixty
days in the hospital, when he would have preferred to stay at
home. No one ever spoke to Don about the possibility of
receiving hospice care, yet according to studies, most people
would prefer to be cared for in their own home if faced with a
life-threatening illness.[1] Unfortunately, like Don, most people
still spend many of their last days in the hospital.

Federal legislation, in the form of the Patient Self-
Determination Act, encourages people to make their treatment wishes known through the use of an advance directive.
Jean did not think Don wanted to be resuscitated, but she
wasn't sure. Don died without having ever discussed with his
family or doctor how he wished to be cared for in the event
that he would face a terminal prognosis. Again, most people
are like Don and do not make a living will or legally identify a
relative or friend to make health care decisions for them if
they are incapacitated.

Compounding the problems brought on by the lack of
advance planning comes recent research reported in the *Journal of the American Medical Association (JAMA)* suggesting that
even when their patient did have an opinion regarding car-
diopulmonary resuscitation (CPR), half of the time the doctor
did not know the person's wishes.[2]

In addition, Don died in pain even though sufficient
technology and the necessary drugs exist to control most pain
in almost all cases. According to the federal government's
Agency for Health Care Policy and Research, cancer pain can
be controlled through relatively simple means for 90 percent
of all patients, yet a statement from the National Cancer
Institute Workshop on Cancer Pain indicated that the
"undertreatment of pain and other symptoms of cancer is a
serious and neglected public health problem."[3]

According to *The Study to Understand Prognoses for Outcomes and Risks of Treatment (SUPPORT)*, half of the patients

able to communicate in the last three days of life said they were in severe pain.[4]

In 1969, Elisabeth Kubler-Ross, M.D., wrote the pioneering bestseller, *On Death and Dying*, in which she said:

> What happens in a society that puts more emphasis on IQ and class-standing than on simple matters of tact, sensitivity, perceptiveness, and good taste in the management of suffering? In a professional society where the young medical student is admired for his research and laboratory work during the first years of medical school while he is at a loss for words when a patient asks him a simple question?[5]

In an editorial accompanying the *SUPPORT* article, Barnard Lo, M.D., writes: "Improving the quality of care generally requires changes in the organization and culture of the hospital. . . . " Lo continues, "Currently, physicians receive little practical training on talking to patients about life-sustaining interventions."[6]

There has been little change in the almost thirty years since Dr. Kubler-Ross first questioned a "society bent on ignoring or avoiding death." It is crucial that we consider options that address the needs of persons with terminal illnesses. Can we care for people at the end of life, rather than just prolonging or precipitating their dying?

Hospice care offers another option to the extremes that many would say are the only alternatives that are available to the terminally ill. Hospice care is a reasoned median between a medical culture that often appears to disregard the needs of the patient and the proponents of euthanasia and assisted suicide who respond to the needs of the dying by offering a premature, medically assisted death.

What Is Hospice Care?

Generally considered a philosophy or program of care rather than a place, hospice is a unique blend of services that addresses the physical, emotional, and spiritual needs of the terminally ill person and his family. Hospice care is provided by an interdisciplinary team of professionals and volunteers, guided by the goals of an individual plan of care. Hospice care emphasizes palliative medicine and supportive services rather than cure-oriented therapies and interventions. In hospice care, the management of pain and symptoms is an appropriate clinical goal and is one of its cornerstones. Services are usually provided in the patient's own home and in such alternative residences as nursing homes, hospice residential facilities, and other congregate living facilities.

The National Hospice Organization (NHO) defines *palliative* as treatment that enhances comfort and improves the quality of the patient's life. No specific therapy is excluded from consideration. The test of palliative treatment in hospice care lies in the agreement by the patient, the physician, the family, and the hospice team that the expected outcome is relief from distressing symptoms, easing of pain, and enhancement of quality of life. The decision to intervene with an active palliative treatment is based on the treatment's ability to meet the stated goals rather than its effect on the underlying disease. Each patient's needs must continue to be assessed and all treatment options explored and evaluated in the context of the patient's values and symptoms.[7]

The Beginnings

The Latin word "hospis," meaning host (and guest), forms the root for the words hospitality, hospital, hotel, and hospice.

It is possible to trace the concept of hospice care back to fourth century Rome, when it was reported that a woman named Fabiola used her own wealth and personal effort to

care for the sick and dying.[8] Later, the Catholic church continued the concept through the Middle Ages by offering a
place of refuge to the poor and sick, as well as to travelers
returning from the battles of the Crusades. These "hospices"
were established to care for ill or weary travelers, and most
certainly cared for the dying.

Dame Cicely Saunders, a London physician, is univer-
sally credited with developing the modern hospice movement
through the establishment of St. Christopher's Hospice in the
town of Sydenham, just outside of London, in 1967. However, the first time the word "hospice" is used to describe a
place to care for the terminally ill appears to be associated
with an institution in France thought to have been established
in approximately 1842, by Mme. Jeanne Garnier.[9] Hospice in
England is known to have begun through the efforts of the
Irish Sisters of Charity between 1885 and 1905, following the
Sisters' efforts to develop hospice care in Ireland in 1879.[10]
Other homes for the dying opened in England during this
period, and one can assume that additional homes were being
established elsewhere in Europe.

Although Dr. Saunders may view herself as simply a
"reviver of an institution originating many centuries earlier,"
her contributions to hospice care establish a clear distinction
between the homes for the dying of the 1800s and what we
now call hospice care. It was the work of Dr. Saunders and
her colleagues at St. Luke's Hospital and later at St. Joseph's
Hospice that led to establishing pain- and symptom-control
as a foundation of hospice care.[11] It was also their work that
led to the use of oral medication, rather than injections,
whenever possible, given on a regular basis to *prevent* pain
rather than to stop pain once it had started. Dr. Saunders was
one of the first to identify the need to address other sources
of pain, and to realize the need to care for a dying patient as a
living person and not simply a dying collection of symptoms.

Dr. Saunders and her colleagues identified the need to
address the spiritual and psychological needs of the dying
person, to understand the importance of the dying person's

family, and to address caregiving through the use of a team of professionals and volunteers.

Two years after Dr. Saunders established St. Christopher's Hospice, Dr. Elisabeth Kubler-Ross, then a physician in Chicago, wrote her landmark book about the end of life. *On Death and Dying* told the story of dying patients and how they wished to be cared for. In the words of a review that appeared in *Time* magazine, Dr. Kubler-Ross's book ". . . vanquished the conspiracy of silence that once shrouded the hospital's terminal wards. It has brought death out of the darkness."[12]

Famous for identifying the so-called five stages of dying—denial, anger, bargaining, depression, acceptance—Dr. Kubler-Ross's work is perhaps more important for identifying three key issues that have been summarized by Charles A. Corr:

1. All who are coping with dying are still alive and have unfinished needs which they may want to address.
2. We cannot be or become effective providers of care unless we listen actively to those who are coping with dying and identify with their own needs.
3. We need to learn from those who are dying and coping with dying in order to come to know ourselves better and to recognize the potential for living.[13]

Almost thirty years ago, dying patients were able to identify the fear that comes from separating them, often unnecessarily, from the support of their own environment. Dr. Kubler-Ross and her patients identified the futility of the ceaseless attempts at heroic measures to prolong life, because such measures so often made dying simply more "lonely, mechanical and dehumanized."[14] Dr. Kubler-Ross's work provided the beginnings of a national dialog on the end of life that is just now gaining critical mass attention.

Hospice Care in the United States

Through the encouragement and assistance provided by Dr. Saunders, the first hospice program in the United States was established in Connecticut in 1974. Established then as strictly a home-care program without the inpatient beds that characterized its model, St. Christopher's Hospice, the Connecticut hospice program itself became a model of care that swept the country. In a very short time, hospice programs were established in Marin, California; Boonton, New Jersey; Boulder, Colorado; and across the country. The Connecticut Hospice, as the first hospice in the United States later came to be known, eventually added inpatient beds and became the first independent hospice inpatient facility in the country.

Today, more than 3,000 hospice programs exist throughout the United States, caring for almost half a million people, primarily in their own homes.[15] NHO estimates that there are more hospices in the United States serving more patients each year than in all the rest of the world. More than 25,000 people work in hospice programs in the United States and as many as 100,000 volunteers contributed more than five million hours of support services and bedside care in the nation's hospices.[16]

Hospice Services

Hospices provide aggressive, comprehensive support and care for persons in the last phases of an incurable disease so that they may live as fully and as comfortably as possible. Prior to the addition of hospice care as a Medicare benefit, the services that a family could expect to receive varied from one hospice to another across the country. Today, a hospice must meet federally regulated operating standards called "Conditions of Participation" to be certified by Medicare as a provider of hospice services.[17] Together with the NHO *Standards of a Hospice Program of Care*, the Medicare certification process for hospices has defined a basic level of service that a patient and family can expect to receive from hospices across the country. (See the resources section of this book.)

Hospice care recognizes dying as part of the normal process of living, so hospice care focuses on maintaining the quality of remaining life. The hospice interdisciplinary team offers a caring community sensitive to the needs of terminally ill persons and their families. With appropriate care, they are free to attain a degree of physical, emotional, and spiritual preparation for death.

Without regard for age, gender, nationality, race, creed, sexual orientation, disability, diagnosis, availability of a primary caregiver, or ability to pay, a hospice program provides comprehensive services to terminally ill persons, their families, and significant others, available twenty-four hours a day, seven days a week, in both home- and facility-based settings.[18]

The typical services that are available in a comprehensive hospice program include:

PHYSICIAN SERVICES

The dying person's personal physician becomes part of the interdisciplinary team of care; however, if the person does not have a doctor, the hospice will provide physician care. Physician services are available on-call twenty-four hours a day, seven days a week.

NURSING CARE

Provided most often through one or more visits to the patient and family each week. As the patient requires, the number and length of nursing visits increase. In addition to nursing care, the nurse also teaches the family how to care for the dying person. Nursing services are also available at all times, whenever needed, twenty-four hours a day, seven days a week.

MEDICAL SOCIAL WORK

Assists the dying person and family with the emotional and psychosocial aspects of the dying process. Additionally, the social worker often assists with problem-solving and with the maze of paperwork that inevitably accompanies a serious illness.

COUNSELING SERVICES AND SPIRITUAL CARE

These services can be extremely helpful as the dying person and his family try to sort out what has now become their lives. How the family comes to terms with the meaning and value of their lives together can impact greatly on their remaining time together, as well as on the lives of the survivors.

CERTIFIED NURSING ASSISTANTS

These aides often provide the most necessary of personal services as they help the dying person and family with activities of daily living. Providing such services as bathing and grooming, the CNA often becomes the closest member of the team to the patient and family.

ADDITIONAL THERAPIES

Hospices provide other therapies—including physical, occupational, and speech therapy—that can be critical to keeping a patient at home. Maintaining one's strength, being able to assist the caregiver when transferring from a bed to a chair, and being able to communicate when no longer able to speak can be very important to maintaining the dying person's control and dignity.

BEREAVEMENT SERVICES

For surviving family members and significant others, these supportive services often start before the death of a loved one and continue for up to a year or more after the death. Bereavement services and counseling are provided on an individual basis and in support groups.

INPATIENT CARE

Although most hospice care is provided in the patient's home, circumstances may arise that make this strategy impossible. Pain and symptoms can become too difficult to be managed at home or the caregiver may experience a crisis. In these and similar circumstances, short-term inpatient care may be necessary. Most hospices provide such care through contractual arrangements with hospitals and nursing facilities; however, some hospices provide such inpatient services directly.

MEDICATIONS, SUPPLIES, EQUIPMENT

Hospices also provide directly or arrange for drugs, medical supplies, and equipment.

VOLUNTEERS

Volunteers provide respite care for the caregiver, spending time with the dying person, reading, talking, and visiting. The volunteer often becomes an important friend to the family by helping with practical needs such as running errands or allowing the family members the time to do these things themselves. Volunteers also can provide important bereavement follow-up and provide critical leadership to the hospice through participation on boards and through administrative or fund-raising work. Volunteers attend an extensive training program prior to working with families.

RESPITE SERVICES

Respite care is available for periods that range from hours to several days on an occasional basis. Respite care can be provided in the home or in a facility.

CONTINUOUS CARE

When necessary, during crisis situations, the hospice may provide ongoing nursing care in the home.

Continuity of Care

Hospice services are guided by a plan of care developed with the dying person and their family to provide a consistent approach to care, regardless of the patient's setting. One of the complaints health care providers hear most often from their patients is that there does not appear to be coordination and communication between the doctors, nurses, and therapists involved with their patient's care in our traditional health care settings. Hospice care, through communication within the interdisciplinary team, responds to this important need for coordination by providing continuity of care across all settings.

Hospice Organizations

While hospice services have become more consistent over the years, the manner in which hospice programs are organized continues to grow in diversity. The largest number of hospices are still independent, community-based organizations. Hospital-owned hospices are the next largest organizational type with home-health agency–owned hospices the third-largest organizational type. Nursing home–based hospices are the least-common organizational type, although the percentage of nursing home–based hospices is rapidly increasing. (See the resource section of this book.)

One of the models for the delivery of hospice care is the Volunteer Hospice Program. Approximately 5 percent of hospices in the United States, found primarily in rural areas, are all-volunteer programs that contract with local home-health agencies or other groups for the provision of nursing and other core services.

Historically, hospices have been primarily not-for-profit agencies; however, as with all health care, there are increasing numbers of for-profit hospices. Currently, NHO estimates that more than 80 percent of all hospices are not-for-profit organizations or—as with Veterans Administration hospices—are affiliated with a governmental agency.

Payment for Hospice Services

Prior to 1983, only a handful of insurers paid for hospice care. In 1982, Congress added hospice care as a Medicare benefit when it adopted the Tax Equity and Fiscal Responsibility Act (TEFRA). The provision was to "sunset" or expire after the third year of implementation, absent legislation to extend the benefit.

In 1986, Congress eliminated the sunset provision, and made hospice care a permanent benefit for those eligible for coverage under Medicare Part A. At the same time, it established hospice care as an optional Medicaid benefit. Today, more than 40 states have established hospice care as a covered service of their Medicaid programs.

The Medicare Hospice Benefit provides coverage of those hospice services necessary for palliation, such as noncurative medical and support services, for a beneficiary's terminal illness. These services must be contained within the hospice's plan of care. The beneficiary continues to use his own physician, who becomes part of the hospice team. The attending physician continues to be paid directly by Medicare if the beneficiary is eligible for physician services under Medicare Part B insurance.

Medicare pays the hospice directly a specified rate dependent upon the type of care given each day. The only cost of those services to the beneficiary is limited cost-sharing for outpatient drugs and inpatient respite care. The Medicare Hospice Benefit requires that the hospice provide bereavement services; however, no payments are made to the hospice program by Medicare for these services. In another departure from traditional Medicare benefits, the hospice is required to provide and document the use of volunteers to augment its services.

Currently, the hospice benefit is divided into multiple benefit periods. The first two benefit periods are ninety days; there is then an unlimited number of sixty-day periods. The benefit periods may be used consecutively, or not.

To be eligible for the Medicare Hospice Benefit, a beneficiary must be seriously ill, with a prognosis of six months or less "if the disease runs its normal course." The attending physician and the hospice's medical director must agree on the prognosis for the patient to be initially certified as eligible for the benefit. The hospice medical director must "recertify" the prognosis of the patient at the beginning of subsequent periods.

A beneficiary may choose to leave the Medicare Hospice Benefit and return to standard Medicare benefits to seek curative care or for other reasons; however, if the beneficiary revokes their benefit during a benefit period the beneficiary will forfeit whatever days are left in that particular benefit period, although they will be able to access additional benefit periods if they choose to again elect hospice care in the future. It is important for the beneficiary to understand that standard Medicare benefits provide less coverage than the service-rich hospice benefit, when used for care of a terminal illness. For example, under standard Medicare the patient is responsible for the full cost of outpatient drugs. Additionally, the beneficiary is responsible for Medicare's usual deductible and coinsurance amounts. A beneficiary receiving hospice care under Medicare may also change hospice programs once each benefit period.

When choosing the Medicare Hospice Benefit, the patient or the patient's legal representative must receive and sign an election form choosing hospice care. This document is essentially an "informed consent" form required of all hospice patients as it describes the nature of hospice services and provides the basis for documenting that the beneficiary chose hospice care. It is particularly important that Medicare beneficiaries complete this document, because when choosing the Medicare Hospice Benefit the beneficiary waives the right to standard Medicare benefits for treatments associated with the terminal illness.[19]

Since its inception, the Hospice Benefit has proven to be enormously beneficial to Medicare beneficiaries as well as hospices. With a stable source of payment, hospice programs have achieved more than a decade of sustained growth and hundreds of thousands of dying persons have been served. Additionally, over the last year of life, Medicare beneficiaries with cancer who are enrolled in a hospice program cost Medicare $2,737 less, on average, than nonusers. This translates into millions of dollars in savings to the government.[20]

Following the development of the Medicare Hospice Benefit, commercial insurers began to offer hospice coverage. It is estimated that more than 80 percent of people with employer-sponsored health plans have a hospice benefit.

Hospice as an Option

In June 1997 the Supreme Court of the United States reversed the rulings of the United States Court of Appeals for the Ninth Circuit and the Second Circuit related to physician-assisted suicide. The Supreme Court unanimously ruled that assisted suicide is not a constitutionally protected right and that the states are free to establish laws prohibiting or allowing the practice of assisted suicide.

This ruling is consistent with the position of the National Hospice Organization as well as most hospice organizations, professionals, and volunteers that assisted suicide should not be legalized. This position is based on the basic principle that hospice care affirms life and neither hastens nor postpones death.

While the hospice community applauded this ruling, it did so because as the debate about assisted suicide returned to the states, the ruling would hopefully allow the discussion to focus on the greater concern of improving end-of-life care rather than on the more narrow issue of whether assisted suicide is a protected legal right. The debate will continue for years.

NHO's studies of assisted suicide suggest that many people support its legalization based on their perception that at the end of life they will be faced with only two bleak options: A death characterized by pain, indignity, and family burden or assisted suicide. Even though hospice answers these concerns, the option of hospice care is not often known to the patient and family or is viewed as an option that should be used only when the patient is on the brink of death. However, NHO's studies have shown that even the mention of hospice care as a more reasoned option to assisted suicide reduces support for the legalization of assisted suicide.

As discussed earlier in this chapter, people have a right to be concerned about the care they might receive from their health care system without the involvement of a hospice. However, for the foreseeable future not everyone will die with hospice support. While demanding that hospice care be more available, we should also insist that all physicians be competently trained in pain management techniques. Additionally, we should require of our medical schools that doctors be taught how to recognize and responsibly respond to depression in their patients. We should also demand that all health care providers be trained in the art of communication so that they are not only capable of having discussions with their patients about the issues of death and dying, but so that they are also capable of communicating their understanding of the patient's needs to their colleagues.

In order to establish ourselves as informed consumers capable of making such demands we must extract a commitment from policy makers and opinion makers, such as the press and entertainment leaders, to understand and value the end of life. These leaders must use their influence to educate rather than frighten and inform rather than confuse.

For example, Jack Kevorkian is generally irrelevant to the discussion of quality end-of-life care; however, the press continually seeks out his comments or those of his legal counsel whenever there is an issue related to end-of-life care. Regardless of how outrageous the comments (or perhaps because of how outrageous the comments), these statements are inevitably shown on the evening news or printed on the front page of our major papers. During the same period of time that Kevorkian has admittedly assisted in the deaths of perhaps fifty individuals, hospices have cared for approximately two million terminally ill people and their families. The knowledge this experience has brought is invaluable, yet telling the public about the hospice story of caring has proved much less appealing to the press than telling the Kevorkian story of assisted suicides.

In 1996, the National Hospice Foundation organized a "media conference" to inform and educate television and movie writers about hospice care. During the conference, Dr. Joanne Lynn talked about how when cultural norms begin to change, those shifts are often reflected and reinforced in the day-to-day lives of our favorite sitcom characters and movie heroes. James Bond now practices safe sex and no one gets into a car anymore on television or in the movies, good guy or bad guy, without putting on their seat belt.

If we are ever to substantially improve end-of-life care, we need to begin to depict death and dying in the same real manner that we show driving a car. We have no trouble depicting thousands of gruesome, violent deaths using every means available from guns to knives to alien spacecraft and exotic viruses, but we seem almost incapable of creating story lines that include death as it usually is for most of us: an inescapable but personal and potentially meaningful part of life.

The Potential of Hospice Care

The growth of hospice care, particularly in the last decade, has been dramatic. Some observers of health care have even expressed concern that hospice care has grown too quickly. However, others have suggested that hospice care serves too few patients.

Perhaps the most accurate view of hospice care is that it is still an emerging form of health care, and its growth cannot be adequately measured using the standards of a mature health care system. Even with the growing awareness of hospice care by medical professionals and the general public and the increase in the use of hospice services, hospice care continues to be underutilized as reflected by the number of patients who are often admitted very late in their prognosis. The average length of stay in a hospice program is approximately fifty-seven days and is even shorter for Medicare beneficiaries. The median length of stay for most hospice patients is shorter still, at approximately thirty days. Fifteen percent of all hospice patients are referred to a hospice within a week or less of their death.[21]

Hospice programs must continue to make access to hospice care a top priority. Physicians need to understand that hospice care provides them another tool to offer their patient, when there is nothing more the physician can do to cure the patient.

Most importantly, the public needs to be informed that

hospice care is not about giving up hope. Hospice care is about courage and hope and about experiencing life. Dying is seldom easy and it requires courage on the part of the patient and the caregiver to face the sometimes enormous physical challenges. And, while hoping for a miracle cure may not be rewarded, hope related to better relationships and to time spent with loved ones can be worth the effort. Life does not end with the determination of a terminal prognosis and dying is not simply a short-term medical event measured in hours and days. The weeks and months that are available to a person at the end of life in hospice care can provide an extraordinary opportunity for spiritual introspection and discovery, an opportunity to express love and to say good-bye.

In his book on early hospice care in the United States, Jack Zimmerman, M.D., wrote "It is important to recognize and accept the fact that the best of hospice care is not going to make every death beautiful and easy."[22] That fact remains as true today as it was when hospice began and it is not the purpose of this book to claim that hospice care is for everyone or to challenge those who will say that hospice care could not help them. Hospice care is a program of services that should be selected only after careful and informed consideration.

In an era of cost pressures and measured outcomes for health care, the value of hospice care involves more than cost savings, and as hospice care is reviewed it may be helpful to consider the words of David S. Greer, M.D., who served as one of the principal investigators in the original National Hospice Study sponsored by the Health Care Financing Administration (1978–1985). In a speech to a symposium of the National Hospice Organization, Dr. Greer remarked that during their study it was not always possible to quantify what they observed in hospice care, but that they were aware that it was something very special.

Chapter Three

SO LITTLE TIME,
SO MANY PEOPLE
A Single Woman Accepts Support

LINGERING IN A cloud of thick confusion and thoughts that wouldn't pass, Anna couldn't believe her fate. How could she be feeling so healthy one day, and within two weeks be forced to take in the news that her life was totally changed? No more work, no more driving, and a future defined only by treatments.

Anna started having strong headaches on a Saturday in late October, and for a few days her left leg felt like it weighed ten extra pounds. By late Monday she was becoming forgetful, even confused, and her speech was slurred. She had a headache that couldn't be eased except by a strong pain medication her allergist had ordered. Even though she didn't want to go, her friends took her to the emergency room at the local hospital on Wednesday. Things happened in a blur after that. There was an MRI (Magnetic Resonance Imaging) and blood work. She was admitted to the hospital that same day.

Anna felt hopeful, and grateful for the medications that brought her relief from her unrelenting headache. At least the pressure that felt like a hand squeezing her brain was gone. Everything was speeding along and she couldn't keep up. There were so many doctors that she didn't remember what they were asking or saying. All of a sudden she was scheduled for neurosurgery on Friday. *I don't want to be sick. I'm only 56,* she kept thinking. Anna felt fear pass through her like a deep chill.

That evening before surgery the members of her women's group and other friends arrived with pizza. Two years before, Anna and her close friend Paula had brought together a group of six women, all with different backgrounds and interests, ranging in age from 48 to 68. They were all close to Anna in some way and their first two gatherings had been supportive evenings that helped her explore different life choices. After the second gathering, the group had decided that the feedback and discussions had been valuable to everyone and they continued meeting twice a month, developing a growing closeness.

Buffered by the attention of her friends, Anna settled into a confident place of believing that the surgeons could remove the intruding tumor from her brain. She wanted to pick up the familiar tune of her life again.

Anna's friends started a chain of phone calls to Anna's family in California and back East and to her friends in town. They notified her supervisor at work about the surgery. Anna's son, Carl, and Anna's sister, Debra, flew in for the surgery, and friends crowded her hospital room. Wrapped in a blanket of concern, Anna felt insulated from the news after surgery that she had a malignant brain tumor, a glioblastoma multiformae. She couldn't remember it all, let alone take in the foreign reality. This was a vicious tumor, one that the surgery couldn't totally remove. Anna's treatment choices were narrow and poor. The oncologist, Dr. Ritter, sat at the bedside and held Anna's hand as he told her in gentle ways about her prognosis. Anna wasn't ready or able to hear the difficult news and continued her cheerful manner. The surgery had removed her symptoms, and physically she felt tremendous relief. She was basking in the care and attention of friends, family, and the hospital staff.

When Anna's son, Carl, her closest friend, Paula, and Paula's husband, Bob, met with the oncologist at the hospital the next evening, he gave them straightforward information that offered some limited treatment options. There was little room for optimism with this type of tumor and the amount of it that the surgeon couldn't remove. As a nurse, Paula had an idea of what to expect. Carl quietly cried as the oncologist described the bleak circumstances.

Three days later, Anna went home. She smiled a lot in those early days, and glowed with the constant visits and calls from friends and family. They were a distraction that kept the cold reality on the horizon. The truth was too large for Anna to take in at that point.

An experienced physical therapist, Anna knew a great deal about health and healing, and believed that she could fight this cancer. She anticipated the six weeks of radiation with positive and calm spirits. Anna's sister, son, and niece returned to their distant homes. Anna had an unusual network of supportive friends and was well loved by many people. Her women's group and her circle of friends visited her, drove her to treatments and doctor's appointments, shopped for her, took care of her finances, arranged for a meal to be delivered each evening, and stayed with her during the first month. For a few nights, Anna said that she wanted to stay alone, but she found that the high doses of steroid medications she took to reduce the brain swelling created anxiety that made it difficult to tolerate time by herself. She described the effect of the steroids as making her feel as though she wanted to crawl out of her skin.

When the next CAT scan X ray was taken after the six weeks of radiation, the remaining tumor was stretching out more. Anna wept as she sat in the oncologist's conference room with Carl, Paula, and Maureen, another friend from the women's group. "I want this tumor to go away," she said. "Aren't there any different treatments we can try? I need to have a chance to fight this cancer. I have a lot more living I want to do." The oncologist, Dr. Ritter, listened and presented other treatment possibilities and options, including chemotherapy. He reassured Anna of his commitment to her care, demonstrating again a compassionate way of telling the truth without destroying all of Anna's hope. He ordered additional medication to manage the relentless, steroid-induced anxiety.

It became increasingly difficult for Anna to be alone even for brief periods of time. When fall semester finals were over in mid-December, Anna's son, Carl, left his third year of university studies, his part-time job, and his two dogs, and came to stay with his mother. It was hard for both Anna and Carl to be together in the condominium again. Anna had moved into the condo with Carl when he was 10, after the divorce. It had been an adjustment for Carl to be in a smaller house, and to be away from his father, who lived back East. During his turbulent adolescence, Carl had always told his mother that he never felt at home there, that he planned to move away as soon as he finished high school. And he did.

Carl still longed for his dad's attention. He felt that the divorce meant that he'd lost his dad. Recently, his dad had remarried and had an infant girl. Carl felt that he was being abandoned, losing both his parents.

Anna felt a strong undercurrent of guilt for needing Carl, for being the one who had to be taken care of in an unfamiliar reversal of roles. Carl wanted to be supportive of his mother, but he resented having to leave his college work and his home. He did not enjoy being back in the town where he grew up, a place he no longer wanted to live. It had taken Carl a few years to discover that he felt more like himself in California; it was his home now.

After discussions with family and friends and consultation at a Second Opinion Clinic at the University Hospital, Anna decided that she would go for one series of chemotherapy treatments. Even though all her research efforts told her she was swimming upstream, she felt that she needed to try everything possible. Every day she took various herbs and vitamins, walked as much as she was able, and focused on therapeutic body work and spiritual practices. Most of all, she wanted to live and have more time.

One of Anna's dreams had always been to go to the ocean to see the annual migration of whales. Since her diagnosis, she had asked a travel agent friend to look into places and costs for such a trip. Now it was clear that she would not be able to tolerate the travel and the stress of the trip. Then there was talk and planning for the women's group to go up to the mountains for a weekend. Even that seemed too much for Anna to consider. Finally, the group made a plan to have an evening gathering and an overnight at one of the member's—Carol's—house, which nestled in the foothills and looked out over the city.

That evening became a special night of sharing dinner, stories, wishes, and remembrances for the group. They made it their adventure and outing together, complete with small gifts, flowers, and treats among the group. In the morning there was breakfast and deer-watching time. Anna said later that while she never got to see the whales, the evening was a delightful substitute. Anna's dreams and plans for the future contracted and shrank as the tumor grew and crowded out her possibilities.

Anna's son, Carl, was feeling overwhelmed emotionally and physically, and the responsibility of caring for his mother felt like too much for him. The women's group set up shifts and stayed with Anna to give Carl more time for himself.

In mid-February, Anna's sister, Debra, came to stay with her for as long as Anna needed. The two women had always been close—"friends, not just sisters," they would say. Anna could relax and felt safe with Debra present. Debra became her touchstone of comfort. A capable organizer, Debra was able to do a great deal of Anna's care. Six years before, when Debra's mother-in-law died of breast cancer, she had cared for her. Debra also nurtured Carl and became part of Anna's special group of friends.

The five women who were part of the women's group that Anna and Paula started were all highly committed to different aspects of Anna's care. Whenever they felt the need, the five of them met to plan and coordinate care, to talk about their fears, frustrations, and limits, and to listen to the difficulties and rewards they were experiencing. Each member of the group had different skills and interests, and they were able to support Anna in that way. One member of the group, Gail, paid Anna's bills and kept track of her finances, (including filing insurance forms) and coordinating help. Patricia called people to arrange for meals. They all brought meals and spent evenings and days with Anna. Sometimes, Debra joined their meetings. The mix of skills and the support they offered, along with the extended circle of friends, made the continuing care of Anna possible.

Anna was touched by Debra's presence, and by Carl's sacrifice in coming to stay with her. There was a constant chain of phone calls, cards, a meal each evening, people to run errands, and other tangible offers of help. It was unusual for Anna to be taken care of, and she worried about being a burden to others. Her anxiety sometimes focused on the toll her illness took on the people she loved. Anna's friends were inspired by her grace and strength in facing all the diminishments of her body and her life. What was most remarkable was Anna's quiet, simple way of asking for help—at one point she said to her son and friends, "I need to be taken care of." And, Anna continued to marvel at the continuing support of family and friends. She basked in the warmth of the visits with the people closest to her.

After the three-day cycle of chemotherapy, Anna grew weaker. As the steroids were cut back, she had less movement in her left arm and leg. She had been using a walker and wheelchair for the past month, but now it was impossible for her to navigate the three flights of stairs in her building. Her friend Bob carried her down the stairs for what would be her final CAT scan and appointment at the oncologist's office.

Again, there was only painful news. Dr. Ritter told Anna, with Carl, Debra, and Paula close by, that the tumor had grown an additional 15 percent in the past three weeks. Anna's weak body sank with the heavy truth. She asked the oncologist, "So, is it time for hospice?" Dr. Ritter nodded and took time to briefly explain hospice services to the family. He reassured Anna that he would visit her at her home, and would continue to be her doctor.

Anna asked what would happen to her in the days ahead. Gently, the oncologist spoke of increasing weakness on the left side, and of sleeping more until she slipped into a coma. He again was firm in his statement that she would have no physical pain. He wrote a prescription in case headaches should occur, and said that the hospice nurse would monitor any and all of Anna's symptoms. Dr. Ritter again reassured Anna that he would continue to visit her at her home.

Carl and Debra met with the social worker in Dr. Ritter's office to make the arrangements for the hospice referral. Paula took Anna outside in her wheelchair. They talked about the terrible news they had just heard.

Paula said, "I hate this. We were supposed to be old ladies together."

"I know," Anna responded. "I don't know what to do. I don't know if I can do this." Paula responded softly, "Well, we've gotten through these past four and a half months—surgery, radiation, and chemotherapy. I suppose we can get through this next part, too. You know you are not going to be alone. Carl, Debra, and I will be here, and the other people who love you will, too. We'll just walk this road together, the way we always have."

"What would I do without you?" Anna replied.

Those were the days when they all cried a lot. Friends from work and from Anna's church continued to bring evening meals for Anna, Debra, and Carl. The depth of caring and support shown to Anna by her friends and family was remarkable. Anna stayed present with quick smiles and as much conversation as her energy would allow. She withdrew only in narrowing down her world and wanting to see just her family, the women's group, and a few others. Anna tried to focus questions on the current interests and activities of her special visitors. Sometimes there were important conversations and reassurances, and sometimes there was just the comfort of sitting together in silence.

For the next five weeks the hospice nurse helped Debra and Carl learn to care for Anna in the shadow of her increasing weakness. A hospice nursing assistant came in five days a week to help Anna to the shower or to bathe her. Paula gave Anna her shower on weekends. Respite aides or nurses were hired three evenings a week so that Debra and Carl could sleep through the night. A hospice physical therapist came in once a week to help Anna with movement and suggestions for maximizing her strength. Anna's weakness progressed so that she needed the support of more than one person to get her long body out of bed.

Several times a week the hospice nurse visited and checked with Anna about her anxiety, about her bowel and bladder function, and about any pain. Gradually, the steroid that reduced the swelling in the brain was decreased, and Anna's anxiety lessened. Each visit the hospice nurse spent time just talking with Anna, and then with Debra and Carl. Typically the nurse stayed for about an hour, examining Anna, answering questions that Anna and her family had, and preparing them for what to expect in the days ahead. She also left a booklet of information about what would happen to Anna physically near the time of her death. At first, Debra couldn't read it, but, she was glad that it was there for later. Debra was strengthened by the hospice nurse's daily phone calls. When Anna's friends visited or called, Debra spoke of how much the support hospice offered was helping.

Since the diagnosis and surgery, Anna had become dependent and endured a constant series of changes and losses. All the people involved marveled at Anna's humor and her lack of complaint over her difficult situation. She wanted to live, and she struggled to understand this unbelievable turn of her life. One week she had to give up lying on the waterbed that she loved and switched to a hospital bed. Her remaining joys were friends and family—and food. Always a tall, thin woman who ate a restrictive diet because of her allergies, Anna now ate, with her oncologist's blessing, any foods that she wanted. She delighted in the surprises of the thoughtfully prepared, sometimes exotic meals friends brought. Each evening a member of her women's group visited at the dinner hour to enjoy the meal with Anna and to help her eat.

Anna seemed to be holding on to life, making valiant efforts to keep up her strength and to be part of the activities of the household. When Debra and Paula talked with her one evening, they asked why she was trying so hard. "Carl's not ready to see me go yet. He still needs me, and we have some things to work through. I guess I need for him to let me know that I can go. I only hope that he will be able to deal with all this."

Stroking Anna's arm, Debra offered, "We'll be there for Carl. He will always be part of our family. We won't let him be alone." Anna sighed deeply and closed her eyes to sleep.

As the days passed, Anna decided to write notes of thanks and good-bye to her family and friends. It was immensely important to her to leave behind written messages of thanks and love for the special people in her life. Her deteriorating vision and tremors in her hands made the fine movements of writing impossible, though, so each morning for the next several days, Debra wrote as Anna dictated the farewell notes. They finished one or two each day, weeping as they did. Debra found it hard to do more than a couple at a time, as did Anna. "It's just so hard to say good-bye to the people that I love. This is the hardest part of it. But I need to do this. It's the last and most important gift that I can give people I love. I want people to know how much they mean to me."

Carl did household chores and errands but still found it difficult to be too close to the care of his mother. He read to her at times and made her her favorite milkshakes. One evening Anna asked Carl how he was doing, and if he thought he would be all right. "I'm going to miss you more than you know, but I think I'll be okay across time," Carl offered. Then he quietly picked up an empty glass and left the room.

While Anna was feeling peaceful most of the time, one Sunday morning she felt impatient, saying she was ready to go. "How many times can you tell people that you love them, or say good-bye?" In a specific conversation with Debra and

Paula, Anna asked whether cutting back the dosage of the steroid would mean the process would happen more quickly. They listed questions for the oncologist, who was planning a home visit on Monday.

When Dr. Ritter visited, he sat down by Anna's bed with his hand on her arm and looked at her as he answered her questions. Together they made a plan to gradually decrease the dosage of the steroids. He reminded Anna that the headaches could return. Later that day the hospice nurse wrote a schedule for decreasing the steroids and made sure the family had sufficient pain medication should Anna begin to have a headache. The hospice nurse told them how important it was once pain occurred to give the oral medications around the clock to prevent a recurrence of the pain. She also put a catheter in Anna since it was extremely difficult for her to get to the bedside commode three or four times a night, as she had been doing.

During the next four days Anna's weakness progressed and she began to sleep more. On Friday she told Paula that she felt foggy, even confused. Paula reassured Anna that her answers were clear and to the point, and that she was tracking the conversation. "The fogginess must just be on the inside for you, because we can't tell it's there." Anna said she was grateful for the feedback and added "maybe my time is closer."

Anna's brother, Dan, decided to drive out since he had promised Anna that he would be with her at the end. The three siblings had become especially close after their mother died fifteen years before. Dan had visited twice before during Anna's illness and he was scheduled to arrive on Sunday morning. On Saturday evening Anna enjoyed what would be her last meal. It was a pleasant dinner, including cherry pie, with Carl and Debra eating with her at the bedside. Dan arrived on Sunday morning. As he sat near her, Anna spoke her last waking words: "Oh, good; Danny's here." Within an hour she slipped into a coma. She was uncomfortable and restless for a short while but a call to hospice brought the nurse quickly to the home, where she showed the family how to give Anna her doses of liquid morphine into her mouth with a small syringe. Anna rested quietly from that point on. The family played Anna's favorite music in the background and lit candles in the room. They tried to create an environment that reflected her style and the things that she loved. The hospice nurse pointed out the decreased circulation in Anna's hands and feet and advised them that Anna would probably only have one or two days more.

All that day and the next, Anna's closest friends visited. There were many tears, remembrances, prayers, and final good-byes. Carl sat for long periods at his mother's bedside, reading and keeping his hand on his mother's arm. Several times he spoke to his mother, telling her that he loved her and wanted her to be at peace.

That Monday Anna died quietly, taking a few breaths just before midnight. Carl called the hospice nurse and Dan called Paula. Paula and her husband, Bob, came quickly and arrived with the hospice nurse. The family members and friends sat with Anna at various points. Carl continued to talk to his mother. Anna's sister, her close friend, and the hospice nurse bathed Anna and dressed her in one of her favorite blue outfits. They talked and prayed together. Two hours later, the hospice nurse called the mortuary and they waited for the funeral director to come, each taking turns sitting with Anna's body. Carl sat with his mother for almost an hour.

Dan, Debra, and Carl stayed in town for another week dealing with the innumerable details that are attached to the death of a loved one. A week later, Anna's memorial service was held at a local church. It was a very personal service that reflected how much Anna was loved. Remembrances by Carl, Debra, Paula, and other friends and coworkers brought tears and smiles to the several hundred people present.

Carl had organized the service and all the arrangements for the gathering afterward at the church. The hospice nurse, and several respite nurses and nursing assistants attended the memorial service and were greeted with warmth and appreciation by the family and friends. The hospice staff members told the family that the experience of working with Anna and her loving extended family was a particularly memorable and special one for them. Later, the family and friends gathered for a meal at Paula and Bob's house and before she left, Debra discretely gave the notes Anna had written to various friends.

Because most of Anna's family lived back East, another memorial service was held there the following week. Anna had chosen to be cremated, so the family took her ashes there to the family cemetery plot. When Carl returned to close up Anna's place, Carl called Anna's women's group and asked them to gather to help him spread some of his mother's ashes. The next day the five women gathered at Anna's, where Carl gave them gifts of photographs of his mother and a special pair of Anna's earrings that she had chosen for each of them. Afterward, they went to the park that Anna had loved and created a ritual where they each sprinkled some of her ashes and said a more personal good-bye. Carl left a week later with a plan to start back to school the next semester and return to his job at the beginning of the month.

Because the family all lived out of town, a hospice volunteer wrote to Dan and Debra back East and to Carl in California. In addition to some written booklets on the grief process, she sent them the phone number of a local hospice program, should they be interested in any bereavement services.

Anna died less than six months after her diagnosis. There was still a sense of unreality about her death for her family and friends. All of them were imprinted by the powerful experience of knowing and caring for her. As Dan said at the memorial service, "The world needs more people like Anna. Her generous spirit graced our lives and will continue to guide and walk with us."

> *When love and skill work together, expect a masterpiece.*
>
> —JOHN RUSKIN
>
> *No one has ever become poor by giving.*
>
> —ANNE FRANK

Caregiving Complexities

Nothing in life prepares us adequately for the demands of caring for someone we love who is dying. Unless you have been involved in the active care of a loved one who is ill and dying, it is almost impossible to imagine what the experience involves. People who are grieving the death of a loved one feel the same way about their reality. Reading about painful encounters, hearing about them, or working with them professionally all offer important understandings and empathy, but they cannot tell us the breadth and depth and the personal impact that living through the caregiving process or the grief process can have. Most people report that the caregiving process and the experience of grief are life-changing events, shattering former assumptions and leading to new ways of being and believing.

Families, like individuals who face life-threatening illness and death, experience a broad range of responses and needs in the strange terrain of illness and death. Our best selves want to be available to the person—to comfort, console, to do all that we can to make the road less difficult and lonely. Those good intentions exist along with our already busy schedules and lives, with very little free time and few spaces. So, no matter how much we love someone and want to care for them in the time of the dying process, the demands can be overwhelming when we try to fit them into our already crowded lives. The emotions and conflicts faced by people who are dying are mirrored in parallel responses by caregiving family members.

Giving care to a loved one means assuming a large measure of responsibility for seeing that their major needs are addressed. Day-to-day life becomes governed by physical symptoms and efforts to ameliorate them. As the person becomes more ill and debilitated, this obligation becomes more difficult and consuming.

Needs of a Person Who Is Dying

There is a distinct set of general needs that have been identified for people who are dying:[1]

1. To be free from pain
2. To retain feelings of self-worth and dignity
3. To receive love and affection

In examining these broad statements of need, it soon becomes clear that they are needs of all human beings. Recognizing common human needs can help us feel less reluctant to be supportive to persons who are dying. First and foremost, people who are facing death are people who are living. The human needs of people who are living with dying are deepened by the power of their experience of illness and by the process of facing death. They experience an intensification and exaggeration of their need for some of the most basic ingredients of life.

Dame Cicely Saunders described the needs of people coping with dying and their family members as

- Comfort
- Control
- Communication

People who are dying have a basic need for physical comfort, as well as for the comforting presence of people who care about them. And in situations where the disease controls so much energy and activity, maintaining some decision-making ability and expressing choices can be immeasurably important. Finally, in times when we feel most alone and afraid, the act of bridging the gaps between people through basic, even symbolic communication anchors us in the safe harbor of shared concern.

The dying process affects people at all levels of their being. This great impact creates the experience of different personal needs as well. All human needs become magnified in times of crisis and stress. The crisis of a life-threatening illness and death also generates a new set of basic needs and emphasizes a higher level of needs related to beliefs and personhood.

Hospice has been defined in its historical form as a "caring community." Part of what hospice offers is a framework, not necessarily a place, for attention to important needs and communication. An important value of hospice care centers around offering people who are dying choices, then working to make those choices possible. Hospice's whole-person, interdisciplinary approach is designed to offer attention to the full spectrum of human needs.

Tasks of Coping with Dying

In addition to addressing the full range of individual needs and responses, current literature on the dying and grieving processes focuses on "task-based models" of coping. These models highlight the individual work that dying persons engage in to meet their situation. The general pattern or framework for looking at the tasks involved in coping with dying developed by Charles Corr[2] follows the recognized dimensions of pain in terminal illness described originally by Dame Cicely Saunders: *physical, psychological, social,* and *spiritual.*[3]

Physical tasks in coping with dying attempt to satisfy basic bodily needs such as physical comfort, nutrition, and rest. Physical distress such as pain, nausea, or constipation is also addressed.

Psychological tasks point to needs around security,

autonomy, and fullness of life. Care that reassures against abandonment, allows for even limited decision-making, and offers a sense of personal dignity concentrates on these important needs.

Social tasks involve sustaining and enhancing significant relationships and facing the social implications of leaving and losing everyone. Many people withdraw from or avoid a person who is dying. On the other hand, the person who is ill decides which people she wants close by and which people she no longer has energy or interest in seeing. Finally, spiritual tasks revolve around identifying, developing, or reaffirming sources of spiritual energy that can encourage faith and hope.

This framework of tasks can guide families as they travel through the maze of difficult emotions, conflicts, and stresses that the process of coping with dying entails. An understanding of these uniquely approached tasks helps hospice professionals collaborate with the family in developing a coordinated plan of care.

Physical Stresses and Needs

In responding to the weight of the demands that are involved in caregiving, there is an urgency around relieving the loved one's physical distress. Hospice care emphasizes the fundamental importance of addressing the physical needs of a person who is dying. The value of palliation or the relief of symptoms cannot be underestimated. In the understanding of human needs, physical needs are the foundation of concern. This primary focus becomes of intensified importance at the end of life, when a disease process is eroding the physical being.

There is no quality of life or participation in meaningful activities when pain or disruptive symptoms are present. One of the romanticized images of hospice care has been of the caregiver or the hospice professional sitting at the bedside holding the hand of the person who is ill and dying. While there is an appeal and a comfort that the image offers, it does not represent the hard physical work involved in the management of ever-changing symptoms that goes on before such an encounter is possible. Mobility, nutrition, and elimination can all be consuming concerns for the person who is ill and for the family members. Only when the physical needs and symptoms are adequately addressed can other important considerations emerge. Family members *do* hold the hands of dying loved ones, but first they expend a great deal of energy and effort giving physical care to the person who is dying.

In a parallel way, the physical needs of caregiving family members can be of the highest importance. Just the simple act of getting an uninterrupted night's sleep is a luxury that some family members go without for weeks or months. Because caregivers are also doing the work and filling the roles of the ill person, exhaustion and irritability are common. Lifting the person who is ill or sleeping on the sofa can create sore backs and chronic muscle aches. Even though family members know that the situation will not go on indefinitely, when you are in the middle of a demanding and in some ways self-denying situation, it can seem to be lasting for an interminable amount of time.

CAREGIVER STRESS RESPONSES

Physical Responses	Emotional and Psychological Responses	Behavioral Responses
Headaches	Irritability	Hyperactivity
Fatigue	Difficulty concentrating	Scattered actions
Neck and back pain	Rapid mood changes	Dependency-related
Complications/	Distancing	behaviors:
recurrences of	Guilt	drug/alcohol use
preexisting conditions	Fearfulness	Withdrawal
Injuries	Depression	Isolation
Sleep disturbances	Anxiety	Decreased functional
Muscular pain		effectiveness
Gastrointestinal		
disturbances		

The major stresses and demands inherent in the caregiving role can leave family members feeling that there is never time to care for their own personal needs or wishes. Some caregivers resent not being able to go for a walk, or to get a haircut, or to have time alone. Caregiver stresses are very similar to the physical, emotional, and behavioral responses seen in professional burnout.

Psychological, Social, and Spiritual Needs

While physical needs are paramount, once they are satisfactorily addressed, other needs emerge under the intense focus of the dying process. The psychological, social, and spiritual needs of the dying person can take on even greater importance as the struggle to deal with the immense reality of death progresses. Hospice care's uniqueness is that it begins with excellent physical care, but, unlike other approaches, does not end there.

Needs and Choices

In many situations, dying persons make choices that may reflect their central concerns beyond their physical being. For example, dying persons often forgo hospitalizations, treatments, or medications that may offer additional time or comfort because of personal decisions they make regarding the quality of their life and the ways that they would like to experience their days.

Anna wanted to have her left-sided weakness and symptoms diminished with the effects of the steroid medications. However, there came a point when the anxiety and side effects that the medication created were less desirable than the advancing symptoms of the tumor growth. By the same token, most dying persons know that hospitals may offer the availability of more vigilant care, and yet most people prefer to stay at home in their own comfortable surroundings, where they maintain a greater sense of personal control. While physical needs are fundamental, they are not the only consideration. Individuals choose to weigh the importance of different needs and prioritize them in a personal way. While it is an important goal to retain the autonomy of the person who is dying, family members may struggle with reconciling their own wishes or choices, which may be different. Hospice care-givers shape their supportive efforts based upon the individual needs, wishes, and ways of coping of the person who is dying, and those of the family members.

Emotions and Responses

In the large constellation of emotions and responses surrounding a life-threatening illness and the death of a loved one, reactions vary in intensity and duration. After hearing the news that her brain tumor was continuing to grow, Anna told Paula, "I don't think I can do this." Typically, we doubt our fundamental abilities to deal with the pressing physical conditions and conflicted emotions that are coloring the situation.

Perhaps the most significant benefit that families discover in their involvement with hospice services is the availability of backup services and consultative feedback that the hospice staff offers. Hospice professionals and volunteers can act not only as support providers but also as buffers against the stresses and emotions that are part of the caregiving process. As human beings, we can find the ability to face painful times if we have around us people who understand the magnitude of the situation and provide tangible assistance to sustain us along the way.

Ambivalence

Even the most loving relationships are colored with ambivalence. For example, parents can feel irritation and dismay with their long-awaited and much-loved infant when he awakens for the sixth time during the night. Caregiving can bring out the dichotomy of love that Khalil Gibran wrote of in *The Prophet*, where love not only brings growth but also involves pruning. It is natural for ambivalence to surface dur-

ing times of great stress, and also when we are in the process
of separation. We want to keep the person close, to stop the
progression of the illness, and we want to be free of the burdens of caregiving. We want to care for our loved one, and we
want a normal life back again.

Resentment and Anger

When someone we love is seriously ill, feelings of resentment
and anger are common. We want the person to be well, to
fulfill the mutual contract of the relationship. We want the
person and our life with them to be the way it has been. Not
only do the changes happen against our will, but they are
counter to our needs.

The act of sacrifice involved in caregiving can generate
feelings of anger and resentment when it is difficult to address
our own needs in a satisfactory way. Anna's son, Carl, struggled
with caring for his mother because he was not ready to have her
die. Anna had always taken care of Carl, and he disliked the
complete reversal of roles. Like most family members, Carl was
angry at the *circumstances* he and his mother were facing. That
anger came from Carl's feelings of being cheated out of time
with his mother and uprooted from his own life.

Another dimension of resentment involves the very real
separation between the large world of a healthy person and
the shrinking world of a person who is ill. Not only is the
loved one unable (or sometimes unwilling) to participate in
the activities and day-to-day events of life, but they may even
resent the fact that others are enjoying life—and they may
communicate that resentment subtly or directly.

Illness can create chasms between people. The person
who is ill is consumed with symptoms and worries about the
unknown future. There is little news except for doctors'
appointments and treatments. It is even difficult to carry on
conversations with people who are seriously ill because they
are out of the mainstream of life, and may not be interested in
world happenings or even the personal experiences of others.

The constant focus on the person who is dying can create an imbalance in the normal rhythm of relationships, where shared interest and mutual concern are expected or needed by family members.

Losses

Responses that seem like envy on the part of the person who is so ill may be an expression of the multitude of losses that a life-threatening illness creates. Beyond physical limitations and changes in the ability to perform even basic tasks, there is a loss of the ability to enjoy day-to-day activities and events. The emotional and spiritual pain involved in a terminal illness creates a sense of separateness and detachment on the part of the ill person that we can interpret in a personal way. The ill person would not want to deny us health or well-being. Rather, she or he longs to be healthy and without limitations.

Regrets

All human relationships involve regrets. We think of things we have had said or done, and wish we could undo them. And we ruminate on the things we wish we had said and done that, for whatever reasons, we couldn't or didn't. By definition, being human means being less than perfect. Death reminds us of lost opportunities and lost potentials.

Guilt

Guilt generated by the impending loss of someone we love can distort the overall nature of the relationship. We forget the private understandings and allowances that all close relationships involve. It is also easy to forget the comforting, healing influence that the passage of ordinary time would have had on our relationships. Many of the difficulties we encounter in our relationships become inconsequential when they are put in the perspective of other day-to-day positive experiences with the person.

While guilt is an almost universal response to loss, spiritual writers distinguish between destructive guilt and true guilt. Destructive guilt is self-deprecating and self-punishing and immobilizes us. Our energy is bound up in blaming ourselves for not being better or different. True guilt recognizes that we have behaved in ways that we do not feel comfortable with, ways that do not fit our sense of who we want to be in the world. This internal realization leads us to resolve to behave differently in the future. In its positive impact, guilt can lead us to a deeper understanding of our values and the principles that we choose to guide our behavior. True guilt carries us forward with the learnings from our past redeemed by the commitment to being better selves in the future. Part of guilt—self-criticism or self-blame—may be an overreaction to the feelings of powerlessness that are imbedded in grief.

One of the many reconciliations that follows the death of a loved one is to see past our deficiencies in a relationship in the framework of the larger picture that also includes all of the positive experiences and moments. Sometimes it is even helpful to play the relationship forward in our minds to see how things would have looked if there had been more time in the future. For example, many of the developmental struggles and discontents that adolescents and young adults in their twenties feel toward their parents melt away with the passage of time. Relationships evolve, and one way to put guilt in perspective is to hold the understanding that, given more time— time we could have naturally expected or anticipated—some of the rough parts of the relationship would have been smoothed out. One of the most beneficial aspects of caring for someone we love when they are dying is the time spent together. Caregiving can counterbalance feelings of guilt and regret that surface after a loved one dies.

Survivor's Guilt

As caregivers, family members and loved ones can experience a kind of "survivor's guilt," the sense of stunned confusion at being near to someone who is stricken, while we are safe and, seemingly, untouched. Our attempts to reconcile the random nature of illness create feelings of ambiguity and loss of control. Along with her family and friends, Anna felt confounded by the fact that she lived a deliberately healthy lifestyle and yet she was facing death from an uncontrollable brain tumor. There are so many questions dying people and their loved ones struggle to settle. Often there are no good answers to those questions, or no answers that satisfy our sorrow.

> Be patient toward all that is unsolved in your heart and try to love the questions themselves like locked rooms and like books that are written in a very foreign tongue. Do not now seek the answers which cannot be given you because you would not be able to live them. Live the questions now. Perhaps you will then gradually, without noticing it, live along some distant day into the answer . . .
>
> —RAINER MARIA RILKE

Powerlessness

Facing our powerlessness is something we don't do naturally or easily, particularly in situations of life-threatening illness and death. In a "solve it," "fix it" world, we want to find answers or do something to ease our discomfort. It is natural to want to find a cause or affix blame in senseless situations or circumstances. Anna did not cause her brain tumor, and she was unable to find a cure. Hospice programs turn the focus toward caregiving as an answer to that discomfort. Echoing Harold Kushner's remarkable words in *When Bad Things Happen to Good People*, hospice workers offer families the opportunity for engaging the questions by moving from asking "Why?" to asking "How can I deal with this?"

Victor Frankl, in his exceptional account of his experiences at Auschwitz, *Man's Search for Meaning*, concludes that we are often unable to control our circumstances. Our only power lies in our responses to those circumstances. Focusing on our distress is important and necessary for a time. After acknowledging the reality that we are in situations that we do not want to be in, we can then begin to draw our map through that strange and fearsome place.

Caregiving Dilemmas

Caregiving creates great inner and interpersonal conflicts. Family members or friends may vacillate between believing that they can do what is required of them in the caregiving role, and then feeling inadequate and incapable of handling the never-ending demands. This "I will do it" versus "I can't do it" struggle is a parallel of the responses that the person who is ill and dying experiences. Both responses are legitimate and are part of the broad spectrum of reactions to a situation where there is such a pressing sense of loss of control.

Avoidance and Involvement

There is a power and magnetism to the realities of everyday demands, like jobs, other family members, and our chosen responsibilities. For the caregiver, it can be comforting to hold to the structure and the distraction that these everyday demands offer for our lives.

An even greater truth is that there is a natural fear and avoidance of people who are seriously ill and dying, no matter how much we love them. It's almost as though we fear the contagion of the illness, or want to keep the person separate, perhaps quarantined so that we will not be touched physically or emotionally by their disease. One of the ways hospice professionals and volunteers model caregiving is in their approach to the person who is ill. By looking at and speaking directly to the person, standing or sitting close, or touching the person gently, family members see that physical closeness can be comfortable and desirable. As with any human reaction or response, the conflict of avoidance versus involvement exhorts us to look at our circumstances and begin to cope with our distress.

Accepting Changes and Limitations

There can be a tendency to take an "all or nothing" position regarding caregiving. Either we take on the full responsibility or we leave it to others entirely. Anna's community of family and friends shared the load of caregiving across time. The friends and family members who had had caregiving experiences set a tone and established a climate where limits were acknowledged and frustrations shared.

Caring for a loved one with a fatal illness is time- and energy-consuming. Anna's sister, Debra, lived out of state, but did not work outside the home at the time. She was willing to leave her husband, her home, and her day-to-day life to be with Anna for the final twelve weeks of her life. It is difficult to juggle the innumerable responsibilities of caregiving with one's own personal commitments. When leaving our own home is involved, especially if distance compounds the situation, it is inevitable that we feel displaced and uprooted. There can be a loss of self in being in someone else's territory, feeling like a stranger with little say about the environment.

Success Versus Rewards

Another source of distress for families caring for their loved ones is the illusion that their efforts could help the person become well again. Just as health care professionals feel frustrated at their inability to offer a cure, caregiving family members feel a sense of futility since the person continues to decline. This lack of a traditional sense of success or reward for our efforts forces family members to redefine their goals.

An additional fear about caregiving involves feeling that either too much will be asked of us or that we will not be able to do what is asked of us. Both are realistic concerns, and both focus on the self, rather than on the person who is ill or the situation. We will never be able to offer all the support for all the need, and if we concern ourselves with fixing or controlling things, success becomes a distant, unattainable goal.

Redefining Healing

One of the foundations of hospice care involves making the goal of care and comfort central, rather than physical healing or cure. The gentleness that Carl showed to his mother in her last days helps us see that there are different levels of healing that are woven into the caregiving and the dying processes. W. Somerset Maugham believed that "the great tragedy of life in not that men perish, but that they cease to love." Anna and Carl did the difficult dance of facing their differences and struggles, while still sharing and appreciating the good moments that were available to them. They both had hoped for more time, and they found ways to make the time they shared during Anna's last weeks as good as it could be.

Anna and Carl turned to others close by to buffer the pain of their separation. Carl talked to Debra about his distress, and turned to friends for support and time away from the intensity of the situation. Anna began to gradually withdraw from her loved ones, becoming quieter and less engaged, except for short periods of time. Perhaps healing for Anna, Carl, and all their loved ones was held in their ability to continue to offer each other caring and love in spite of all the difficulties and the natural self-protective inclinations that could have pulled them away from one another.

Offering and Receiving Support

Support is a global, inclusive word, like love. While it may be difficult to define specifically, there is an undeniable sense of caring that is inherent in the experience of offering and receiving support. A definition of genuine support includes three dimensions: *respect for one's autonomy, compassionate concern,* and *regard for the person's ability to function independently.*[4] The offering of support involves filling in the aspects of need that the individual is not able to provide for him- or herself. Supporting people facing difficult times does not involve taking over and making decisions for them.

There are no universal formulas for supporting people who are facing death and grief. Each individual and family meets the painful times of their lives in the context of their particular history and beliefs, their personality and the strength of their relationships. It takes effort to bridge the emotional, social, and spiritual pain that isolates people who are dying and their family members. The act of offering support and care to another involves extending ourselves and being present. People can't know of our concern if we keep it in the realm of good intentions. All of us have regretted the call we didn't make, the condolence note we never wrote, or the funeral we chose not to attend.

For example, a young woman was struggling with a severe upper respiratory infection when her grandmother died. She visited her family physician and asked if she was well enough to travel by plane to her grandmother's funeral. The physician, knowing the woman had recently been separated from her husband, saw that she was unsure about whether or not she wanted to go to the funeral, whether or not she felt up to it emotionally. Without pressure, the physician told her, "I can give you some medication that will make you feel a bit more comfortable. You would be well enough to travel, if you wanted to. It's important to remember that you don't redo a funeral. So, if you decide not to go, you may ask yourself whether you would regret it later on." That simple reminder that funerals are one-time opportunities to say good-bye helped the young woman decide to travel to the ritual. Support frequently involves reaching out past our own concerns and being available when it would be easier not to do so.

Sometimes we stay away from people in painful times of their lives because we worry that we don't have the stamina or ability to be with them. We are self-conscious about saying or doing the right thing or we're afraid that the personal price of offering support will be too high. For more than six months, Anna's community of family and friends stayed with her and were irrevocably touched and changed. Each of them learned invaluable lessons about the nature of caring and supportive relationships.

What is needed most is for us to stand with people in the face of their dying and grief. Hospice professionals and volunteers work to create opportunities for being together that reflect the needs of people who are dying and of their loved ones. It is an experience of the best in us as human beings that imprints everyone involved with its power and sacred memory.

... When we honestly ask ourselves which persons in our lives mean the most to us, we often find that it is those who, instead of giving much advice, solutions, or cures, have chosen rather to share our pain and touch our wounds with a gentle and tender hand. The friend who can be silent with us in a moment of despair or confusion, who can stay with us in an hour of grief and bereavement, who can tolerate not-knowing, not-curing, not-healing and face with us the reality of our powerlessness, that is the friend who cares.

—HENRI J. M. NOUWEN
Out of Solitude (1974)

Chapter Four

MY LITTLE ONE
A Mother Remembers
Her Baby's Brief Life

June 24

This time in my life should have been one of the happiest times, and instead it's like a nightmare. I'm 29 years old and three days ago I gave birth to my first child, Joseph. Ron and I were ecstatic to be having our first baby. I went into labor three weeks early, and there was some concern because Joseph was in distress during the delivery. His body looks beautiful, even though he is small at three pounds, two ounces.

After doing a number of tests and X rays these past few days, the doctors told us yesterday that our Joseph will not live more than a few weeks. I feel numb, even though I have not stopped crying. I hear the words that the doctors have said, and I know they would not tell us such unbearably cruel news if it weren't true. I don't want to believe it.

My husband, Ron, kept saying to the doctors, "There must be something you can do. Why won't an operation fix his heart?" Because Joseph's condition is inoperable and even a transplant wouldn't be possible, they suggested we could keep him in the hospital or take him home. I want to take Joseph home more than anything. I'm so afraid. I decided to write this journal to have a way to help myself deal with this, to calm myself. And if Joseph's life is going to be so short, I want to remember everything that I can about him, and about our time together. Because I will need to focus on caring for him, this will be a place to put my tears.

There are so many plans we need to make to bring Joseph home. The nurses said they would show me some of the things that would be helpful for me when I'm caring for him. Sue, the social worker, recommended hospice. She told me hospice had worked with a number of families in similar situations and had been very supportive to the parents. I had never heard of hospice, but I was sold when she told me that they would do everything to help us take care of Joseph at home. Ron will help, too. We just don't know how much time they will let him take off from work. Now that the decision is made to take Joseph home, I can't wait until tomorrow. There is a part of me that thinks when we get him home, we can love him enough so that he can be okay. I still can't believe that this is true. I don't want it to be true.

June 25

It's 5 A.M., too soon to go to the hospital. I'm so anxious to have Joseph home. Every moment seems important. The hospice nurse will meet with us in Joseph's hospital room at 10 A.M. After we make all the arrangements and the nurses teach me some special feeding techniques, we will come home.

I realize that I am only thinking about Joseph living, not about his dying. And I suppose that every minute he lives he is dying. Ron and I agreed last night that we won't pretend. We're going to try to enjoy Joseph and show him as much love as we possibly can in the time that we have. That's not hard to do since he's such a sweet baby, with his soft brown hair and his perfect features. He has Ron's face, but my coloring.

June 26

Both Joseph and Ron are sleeping, and I'm up early again. We have Joseph in our room at night, in his bassinet. I woke up this morning and didn't hear Joseph breathing for a few long seconds. I panicked until I heard him. Then I went to look at him, so small and vulnerable. I want to hold him close every minute.

It wasn't too difficult to bring Joseph home yesterday. It just seemed strange to be talking with the hospice nurse, Sandy, so calmly about Joseph's condition. She called the house late yesterday afternoon and will come by this morning. I think I'm going to like her. Quiet and low-key, she also seems very warm and competent. I'm especially relieved about the 24-hour on-call services. Having someone to call if I need to is reassuring to me.

I know that I'm pushing this painful reality away. There is a numbness I feel around the truth of Joseph's condition. Out of the blue today I felt a sharp terror about what I will do when he gets weaker, or when he dies. Then I talk to myself and tell myself that all I need to think about is the present, this day we're facing now. I'll try to use the Scarlett O'Hara approach to worrying about the rest tomorrow.

June 27

I'm amazing myself with my mothering. I seem to be handling Joseph's care and keeping my fears at bay. Joseph is so tiny that both Ron and I worry about hurting him. Sandy has been wonderfully helpful with all her practical suggestions. I told her yesterday that to be a hospice nurse you must need to have a great deal of experience, and a lot of common sense to go with it. She has a way of being very clear-sighted, reminding me of what's important and which things I should not focus on too much. It's important that Joseph drink small amounts more frequently, but I shouldn't worry if he goes a bit longer without eating, or doesn't take in much. I'm learning to trust Joseph and to trust my own mothering instincts.

When I began this journal I decided not to talk about the medical facts of Joseph's congenital heart defect. Actually, Ron is the one who's been doing the research, making the phone calls to specialty clinics and keeping all the medical records. He's been recording Joseph's pulse, respirations, and color in a log that he keeps for Sandy and Dr. Evans, our pediatrician. It's his accountant personality to want to quantify, measure, and solve things. I wish that Joseph's heart was repairable. His tiny body is such a wonder to me that I can't imagine that he has a heart that isn't going to be able to keep him alive.

I don't understand how this could have happened. I was at the pinnacle of my health during this pregnancy, and I thought that I did everything right. There have never been any type of birth defects or congenital problems in either of our families. The doctors have given us all the answers that they have, and recommended genetic counseling later.

In some ways, this journal is my collection of memories about Joseph. I want to remember Joseph and how we are together as a family. We're taking lots of photos, too. Already I can't imagine how I will be able to let him go. Every time that I write, I end up crying.

June 28

Joseph sleeps a lot and doesn't have a great deal of energy. There is a softness about him that makes me want to hold him all the time. Sometimes I do just sit and hold him and sing to him as he sleeps. Yesterday I started singing "You are my sunshine, my only sunshine" to him. It's a song my mother always sang to me. When I got to the line "please don't take my sunshine away," I cried and cried. I would beg, plead, bargain away my own life with God or anyone who could save my son from his terrible fate.

If I let out some of my sorrow in this journal, it leaves me sad and depleted. That's what happened yesterday. I almost didn't want to write today, but I also realized that once I look at what's happening to us, I feel more able to handle it. At least I'm aware of what's going on inside me. I don't want my sorrow to spill over on Joseph and Ron all the time. This is a better place for it now. I keep struggling to balance out the beauty of Joseph's presence here with us against the piercing fact that he will not be here for very long.

Joseph is one week old today. Last week at this time I was giving birth. So much has happened in this week that I can barely take it in. I seem to have a need to try to keep up emotionally with things. I need to know the truth about Joseph, and I wish that this terrible truth was a mistake. I want to feel, and yet I don't want to feel too much sorrow now. Sometimes I just push things back so that I can be with Joseph. Everything inside of me is in turmoil.

Family and friends are calling, though we have discouraged people from coming to the house. The doctors warned us that Joseph has very little immunity, and any infection could shorten his already brief life. I also don't feel like socializing much with other people. I want to focus on Joseph and Ron. My parents will be driving out from Springfield in a few days. They told us they wanted to meet and know their only grandson. Ron and I thought that it would be important for us to share Joseph with them. We get along well with my folks, and they will be a help when they're here. Ron will probably go in to work for a few days.

There are times I feel like a little child, wanting to sit and cry, wanting someone to hold me for the longest time and make this better. I'm afraid of how I will be when Joseph dies. I'm worried that I won't be able to survive this heartache.

June 29

Eva, the hospice volunteer, came to visit today. She's 71 and exudes kindness. She brought homemade chicken soup and listened while I talked. Then she straightened out the kitchen before she left. It wasn't difficult to have someone who was a stranger come into our home at this time. I thought that it might be, but Eva responded in her gentle manner to all the things that I suggested.

Joseph is tracking more now. He seems to look directly at me with such knowing eyes. I asked him questions today when I held him. "Do you know how much I love you?" "Are you uncomfortable?" "What would you have enjoyed as a little boy?" "What am I going to do without you?" I love holding Joseph, and I never want to put him down. Sandy, the hospice nurse, says it's fine to hold him as much as I want. He sleeps in his own bedroom now. There's just more room in there. When he's asleep in his bassinet, sometimes I pull over the rocker and just sit stroking him, or holding my fingers over his tiny hand.

I've gotten into the habit of singing to Joseph, and of playing the music box that sits on his dresser. My sister sent it before Joseph was born. It plays "Edelweiss," and I love humming along. Recently, I've replaced my own words for those in the song. "Soft and sweet, our heart's delight, bless our Joseph forever." I had to change the line "may you bloom and grow" because I know that Joseph never will.

So many things set off my tears. It's strange what will trigger them. Yesterday I got a card from my friend Barbara. We've been friends since the first grade. I remember when her mom died during our senior year in high school. We became even closer after that. She wrote such a caring note in the card, and offered to fly out if I wanted her here. It wasn't the words that she wrote that touched me; it was picturing her writing them, and knowing that I could count on her in difficult times. She told me that she had cried for me, for Ron, and for Joseph when she heard the news. That's when I started crying. Once I do cry, then I can go on again for a while. I'm beginning to realize that I need to cry. This is the saddest thing that I could ever imagine happening. If I can get through losing Joseph, I know that I will be able to survive the other losses in the years to come.

June 30

It's the end of June, and this is the month of Joseph's birth. July will most likely be the month of Joseph's death. I tell myself not to think things like that, but the thoughts come of their own accord. I'm trying to just look at them, and then let them pass without dwelling on them. So far, that seems to work.

Ron went to work today, so everything seems busier. He'll work a half-day today and tomorrow; after my parents arrive, he'll work for the rest of the week. We're taking it one week at a time, actually one day at a time. I'm relieved that the people at work have been understanding. Ron's boss told him that he could take time off, but that he did want him to keep up with a couple of accounts. So, he's trying to do that.

More people are calling now. Our pastor wanted to come by this week, but I asked him to wait and come out when my parents were here. That way if I don't want to visit with him, my parents can speak with him. Two coworkers called this morning, and I realized that I didn't want to speak with them. I told them I needed to go feed Joseph. Eva came by this morning and she answered phone calls while she was here. I like having Eva around. I know it's because she is so easy to talk to, and she has a calming influence on me.

Joseph has been stable, with few changes. Since he was born, he has only gained one or two ounces. Today I noticed more blueness around his mouth, and he seemed listless. Sandy, our hospice nurse, is scheduled to visit three times a week. Eva suggested that I call her since I was worried about Joseph. An hour later Sandy came, and she noticed the changes, too. We talked about the fact that the blueness may come and go, and that Joseph was still stable. I'm aware that this time is so important, and it seems to be passing so quickly. Every day that passes means that Joseph's life is growing shorter. I will be glad when my parents arrive. I feel shaky and alone today.

July 1

I will never forget how excited my parents were to see Joseph. They were as proud as any grandparents I have ever seen, and cried mostly with happiness. My dad held me for the longest time when they arrived, and I clung to him as if I would crumble if I let him go. I had no idea how relieved I would be when my parents arrived. They have always been so stable and supportive. In spite of all their little faults, I realized how much I needed them here, needed their solid love. It was also wonderful to have more family to love Joseph, to know him and treasure him the way Ron and I do.

Joseph was awake a little more today. Maybe he picked up on all the excitement. He focused his striking blue eyes on each of us, forming a connection that held us close to him. Ron and my dad took a lot of pictures, and it felt like the first real celebrating we've done since Joseph's birth. This was a happy, good day for all of us, a day I know I will never forget.

July 2

Mom and Dad are out shopping for groceries. They will start cooking and doing every possible helpful thing they can think of for us. Dad already cut the lawn this morning, borrowing the neighbors' push mower so he wouldn't wake Joseph. It was one of the things that Ron just didn't get to. I realize how good it is to have someone just pitch in and do things that need to be done, without being overbearing.

I feel less afraid today, though sleep is still difficult. I'm always listening for Joseph's breathing on the baby monitor. Mom got up with me once last night and just watched and listened to me talk about our routine, about Joseph's condition.

July 3

When the stores opened, Dad took all the film in to be developed, and now we have wonderful pictures. Joseph looks so tiny, but he is awake in almost all of them. Eva came by and helped Mom send them out to family and friends this afternoon. Mom and Dad like Eva as much as we do, and enjoyed talking with her. Later, Mom said that it was good for them to have someone to talk to, so that they could be as supportive as possible to us.

July 4

It doesn't seem like a holiday today, and I can't seem to relate now to the idea of freedom. The five of us are here, and that's special. I'm glad that Ron is home today and for the rest of the week. I noticed that Ron got quieter, almost more depressed those days that he worked. He said that it was difficult for him to concentrate at work, but he did update the accounts that were pressing. Being with Joseph has brought us closer together, though we don't talk much about losing him. We can't always defer or push the sadness back, but most of the time we just stay close to Joseph and each other.

Joseph grows sweeter each day. My day centers around him, caring for him—holding him, or just watching him. Mom and Dad seem to understand completely the need I have to be near him. Their presence has helped more than I imagined. It's good not to have to think about meals, or laundry, or even answering the phone.

In addition to keeping this journal, I've been praying. At first I prayed that this reality would not be true, that Joseph would live. I still wish that one morning we would get a phone call from the hospital saying that there was a new procedure that would save

Joseph. So, I pray for a miracle. More than anything in the world I want Joseph to live. Every day I see his weak and frail little body, and I know that I need to pray for my own strength to handle this.

Joseph is teaching me so much about love. I never knew what it would be like to put someone else first. That's not to say that I don't love Ron. He grows dearer to me all the time, especially given how caring and loving he has been through all this. He's been such a tender and strong daddy to Joseph. Being a parent is a sacred experience, one that has made me a bigger person, and has taught me to rise above my own concerns to care for Joseph. Will I still be a mother when Joseph dies?

July 5

When Sandy came today I felt like she was raising a warning flag about Joseph's condition. He is getting weaker, and she reminded us that he would sleep more and eat less as the days went on. It was difficult to hear, but it helps that we know what to expect. There are moments when I forget, and this doesn't seem real. When I see Joseph sleeping, I think he is a normal baby, and this has just been a bad dream. I wish that I could awaken and find this not our true situation. I felt a huge flare of anger today. Why are we all being cheated out of time together?

Seeing that I was upset, Sandy asked if we would be interested in a visit from our pastor or the hospice social worker. My immediate response was "No," but I told her we would think about it. Religion is the furthest thing from my mind right now. Later on I will have a lot of sorting through to do about my faith, and how I see God. How could God let this happen? I'm too angry to look at it now.

July 6

Joseph, our tiny angel, is weak but still fairly stable. I did hear what Sandy was saying yesterday. Things could and will change anytime soon. When I rocked Joseph this morning after his small feeding, I talked with him, asking him to fight as much as he could, so we could have more time together. I keep telling him how much I love him. Whether or not he understands the words, I know he can hear the love in my voice. Last night I realized that we probably never have enough time with someone we love deeply. It's too difficult to write more today.

July 8

I felt immobilized yesterday, and unable to write. The weight of reality was so heavy that I felt like I was moving in slow motion. I'm relieved to have Mom and Dad here. They are helping so much, doing all the tangible things to keep the house running, caring for Ron and for me, and spending sweet time with Joseph, too. I don't know what I would do without them here now.

Joseph is sleeping more, and I notice he makes fewer movements with his hands. His eyes are so expressive, though. I could look at them for the longest time, and when I do I'm talking and singing to him. Is it my imagination that he is responding less? He seems so weak and tired most of the time. I wish that I could infuse my spirit and energy into him. I would give him my life if I could. And how I wish that I could.

July 9

My sister, Laurie, wants to come out for a weekend. And Ron's father wants to come and meet Joseph, too. I want them to come, and yet I'm worried about too many people being here, and that I won't have enough energy to keep up with the demands. I'm also aware that every day our time grows shorter. I want to spend every possible minute with him. Ron does too. He's decided he won't go back to work while Joseph is still here. I'm so relieved for all of us that he will be here, that we'll all be together for the days ahead.

My mother arranged to sleep at our friends, the Warners, with Dad for the weekend. That way Laurie can have the spare room and we can all have some time to visit. She's coming out this weekend. We have always been close, and I do want her here.

Nothing seems right to me. I feel irritable at times, and then I feel physically hit by the truth and I want to howl like a wounded animal. I've always thought that the coyote's howl sounded like a song of wanting, of longing. What am I wanting and longing for? Joseph, more time with Joseph.

July 10

Our pastor called and came to visit today. Mom and Dad said that they would like to meet him. I visited in on their conversation at a couple of points, and found it to be a gentle exchange, with lots of understanding on our pastor's part. He seemed very caring. My fear was that he would come and preach religion and "God's will." I can't imagine that God would want Joseph to die, to be so weak and frail, to have so little time.

Mom said he asked them what questions they were struggling with, and they told him how they just couldn't comprehend or understand this innocent child dying. When I sat in, I told the chaplain that I didn't feel that God caused this tragedy, but I wondered how he could just stand by and watch it happen. It makes me too angry if I think about that piece. We spoke about the random nature of the universe, and the irreconcilable nature of situations like Joseph's. He said that God understood our suffering and loved us through it. I wish I could believe that. I feel very abandoned by God at times.

Mom and Dad see their faith as a comfort they can hold on to, and they believe that we will all see Joseph again. I don't know what I believe now. And seeing Joseph again sometime in a vague, distant future does not feel like enough. I want him here with me, to grow up with Ron and me loving our son until we are old and ready to leave. That's the way things are supposed to happen.

July 11

Each day Joseph slips away just a little, eating less, moving and responding less, and sleeping more. We still hold him a great deal, probably eighteen to twenty hours a day. None of us can get enough closeness with Joseph. Yesterday when I saw my dad walking the nursery holding Joseph and talking to him, I cried. My dad never had a son, and now his first grandchild, the long-awaited boy, will be gone soon. When I think of all that we will miss with Joseph, all the times we won't have with him, then I get overwhelmed with the loss. We're not just being cheated, we're losing all the promise and potential that a baby brings to a family. I'm sad for Joseph, for Ron, for our family, and most of all for myself. I want Joseph with us, with me. I don't want him to die.

July 12

Joseph had a restless night, and Sandy came out to check him this morning. She told us that the inability of Joseph's heart to function is almost cumulative, creating more decline as the days go on. She reassured us that he would not die today, but that his time was growing short. I knew it was actually happening. I just didn't want to admit it to myself.

During the night, when Ron and I were taking care of Joseph, trying to comfort him, I told Ron that I was afraid that the end was coming soon. It helps when Sandy tells us what to expect. She told us that Joseph wouldn't be crying much these next few days, because he wouldn't have the strength. All that is left for us to do is try to keep him as comfortable as possible, and to love him. We will never be able to show him all the love that we feel. I believe that he knows me, and Ron, and he seems to be peaceful and content. Those are small parts of parenting, but they mean a great deal to both of us.

Ron cried today when Sandy was here. It's starting to hit him now. We seem to seesaw back and forth with our sorrow and our need for support from each other. It helps that my parents are here. They truly have been taking care of both of us.

My sister, Laurie, arrives later this afternoon. She's always been strong and able to handle a crisis. I'm glad that she will know Joseph, though he seems less himself now, and so fragile. Ron's dad arrives on Sunday, the day that Laurie leaves. Our neighbors brought in a daybed that they put downstairs in the recreation room. It seems right for everyone to stay here with us.

July 13

Joseph is the same as yesterday, with less restlessness during the night. We took shifts of two hours each holding him during the night, and we were all more relaxed. He seems better when we hold him, so we will keep on holding him as much as we can. It wasn't difficult to share him with Ron and the family today. It feels like we're all so close together with this experience. I'm glad that I won't have to explain to everyone about what Joseph was like. He is achingly precious to us.

Laurie loves Joseph, and she's wonderful with him, and with us. She has brought more love and caring into the house. It all helps. When there are people who love us around there is less pain. Maybe the love counterbalances it. It doesn't take the sadness away, it just makes it bearable.

I tried to take a nap this afternoon, but I couldn't fall asleep, as tired as I was. Laurie brought me a book, *Anna: A Daughter's Life*. At first I didn't even want to look at it, but then I picked it up off the nightstand. I told Laurie that I was writing a journal about Joseph and our experience. The book was written by William Loizeaux, a father whose first child, Anna, was born with congenital defects, too. When I flipped open the book, the first passage I saw talked about how some of his best memories of Anna were seeing her in the arms of others. That's very true for me. I'm anxious for Ron's dad to arrive tomorrow. Since Ron's mother died six years ago, before Ron and I met, it must feel doubly sad for them with her gone, too.

I put the book down after that. That little piece I read, almost a confirmation of what is happening here now, was enough. My tolerance is not high. So I closed my eyes and tried to rest, but couldn't. Too many thoughts and feelings were floating through my mind, like clouds in fast-forwarded film. I could barely see their form and shape before more replaced them. I got up and went to the kitchen and sat with Ron, Dad, Mom, and Eva, the hospice volunteer. I'm surprised at how well Eva and my parents get along, like they're old friends. I joined Laurie in Joseph's room, where she was holding him and humming one of our favorite old Beatles songs. It struck me how much we had shared across the years, and I wondered how my life would have been without Laurie for a sister. If Ron and I are able to have any other children, their lives will be poorer for not knowing their brother, Joseph.

July 14

Joseph is sleeping more, and he seems hungry at times, but doesn't cry. Today he's making a muffled sound that is more like a whimper. He doesn't take much milk, even with the little dropper we use. A nipple is too much work for him. When I let myself take this all in, I realize that he can't last much longer.

Last night when we were in bed holding each other, Ron talked about his mother's long struggle with breast cancer, and how painful it had been to live through those three years of surgery, treatments, recurrences, and progressive illness. "It was like seeing her become diminished as time went on. She had such a positive outlook, and tried· so hard to be well. Nothing worked. There were parts of it that feel a lot like what is happening with Joseph. Only then I was in high school and starting college, and I kept my distance from most of it. I· never believed that my mom would die. It was one thing for her to be sick and weak from the radiation and the chemotherapy, but I never dreamed that they wouldn't work. I sometimes think that the odds are against me. There's never been a good break when someone I love has been sick. It always turns out in the worst possible way."

I didn't know what to say, so I just held him tight and told him how much I loved him, how glad I was that we had found each other. One of the hardest parts of this is watching the people that I love grieve. It makes me feel powerless and amplifies my sorrow. Sometimes there's so much sadness inside me that I don't know what to do with it, where to put it.

July 15

I didn't want Laurie to leave yesterday. She cried for a long time when she was holding Joseph and saying good-bye, and soon we were all crying. I know she will come back for the funeral, but I can't even think about that now.

Ron's dad arrived late yesterday morning. I could see and feel the relief and sorrow in Ron. When I see him with his dad, I see two men with a bond that has been made deeper because of losing someone they loved a great deal. That will probably happen again with Joseph.

I wish Ron's dad had come sooner. He's stepped right in and become an easy part of the family as we all care for and love Joseph and each other. Joseph seems to be slipping further away now.

When Sandy made her usual visit today, she spent time with Ron and his dad, and with my folks, answering their questions, giving them an idea of how she saw Joseph. It seemed like they talked for more than half an hour. I decided to stay with Joseph. I seem to bounce back and forth with how much reality I can handle. For today I just want to spend time with Joseph and not think about things too much.

July 16

Ron is more worried about Joseph losing ground. He told me it was hard not to feel like he should be doing something. We both feel so helpless, like a huge storm of threat is coming toward us slowly, and we can't do anything but stand by and watch it prepare to punish us with its terrible force. I want to scream "No!" and "Stop!," but the sound is caught with all the tears in my throat.

I had a nightmare last night, but I only remember a few images. They've haunted me all day. I'm walking down a long path, alone, looking for Joseph, and I can't find him. Everything is foreign and foreboding, and I keep trying to find him, or to get someone to help me find him. I'm running and become more and more frantic as time passes. Then I woke up, in a panic. I don't often remember my dreams, and this one is clear and obvious in its message. I *do* feel panicked at losing Joseph.

July 17

Yesterday my mother told me that Sandy had asked if we would like to call the funeral director to make arrangements. I can't do that now. My mother asked which funeral director we would choose, and said that Ron's dad would call and tell them what we would be wanting. It felt like a good compromise, and Ron and I did not have to deal with it now.

All my energy and attention is going to Joseph. He's breathing with more difficulty now, and is barely responsive. Sandy is coming every day, and asked if we would like the hospice social worker to come by and talk with us. I can't deal with anyone new at this point, and this is not the time for talking. It's the time to be with Joseph while he's still here with us.

July 18

We're losing Joseph. He just can't seem to hold on much longer. Sandy was here for a long time this morning. She said Joseph probably would not make it through the day. I still can't believe it. Ron's holding him now. A part of me is holding tight to the belief that if we hold him and sing to him we can keep him alive here with us. It's unbearable to watch him slow down to the point where he's barely able to breathe, and he hasn't taken anything to drink for the last eighteen hours. His little hands and feet are cold and blue. I keep repeating to myself that this can't be true.

July 19

Joseph died at 10:30 last night. We cried for several hours, as he was dying, and afterward. I feel like I'll never stop crying for Joseph. My heart is so heavy and my arms are frozen and empty.

Joseph just kept fading away, as if you could see his body slowing to a stop and his spirit leaving. I was holding him when he died, and Ron was encircling us both, stroking Joseph's hair. Mom and Dad, and Ron's dad and Sandy, were there with us. Even after our Joseph was gone, I didn't want to put him down. We all took turns holding him and saying our good-byes. Sandy said we could wait as long as we wanted to call the funeral director. Neither Ron nor I wanted to let him go. Finally, in a span when our tears were subsiding a bit, we told Sandy to call, and they took Joseph at about 2 A.M.

The house is so empty now, even with all the phone calls. I realize how much Joseph's presence kept me going, how he was the focus of everything. Now that he's gone the void is almost unbearable. Ron and I have been leaning on each other, and on our family. Our lives are so much less without Joseph.

Eva came this morning and helped orchestrate the schedule and details of the day. I'll be glad when Laurie gets here this afternoon. Our minister will be by tomorrow to help with planning the service. Ron and I will go with his dad to the mortuary to finalize the arrangements. He wanted to do that with us, and he is very practical and grounding in his manner. I know that he will let us make our own decisions. I don't want to be doing any of this. Ron is holding up, but he seems so weary and burdened by all the sorrow. I don't know how we're going to be able to face the funeral on Monday.

July 20

There seems to be a flood of calls, flowers, cards, and food. Some close friends have come by to the house, bringing hugs and kind words. I feel out of my body sometimes, unable to feel things or take them in. Ron says he feels that way, too. It's good to have distraction because all I want is to have Joseph back. I can hardly bear to walk past his room. Ron closed the door, and I'm not sure if that feels right either. Nothing is right with Joseph gone.

Tomorrow is the funeral, and I don't know how I will face seeing his tiny casket at the service. What I dread most is the cemetery. How do people live through these unbearable moments? I wonder if I can, and then I think that I don't want to. Not that I'm suicidal. It's that staying alive when Joseph is dead is difficult beyond my imagining. I want to be with him, or more, I want him back here with us.

July 22

There was no time or energy for me to write yesterday. The funeral had some comforting and some painful parts. We chose to play Eric Clapton's song, "Tears in Heaven," and I lost my composure when it played. I will never forget the image of Joseph's small casket in the church, or of the cemetery. Leaving him at the cemetery was excruciating. I had all these horrifying images of his beautiful body in the casket being put into the ground. I forced myself to stop thinking about it because that image seems destructive.

Joseph would have been one month old yesterday. I thought about that at the funeral. How can we be burying our son who wasn't even a month old?

How can life go on for the rest of the world? How can the sun shine so brightly, and everything look so rich with summer green when Joseph is dead?

Mom and Dad will stay for another week. Ron's dad will leave on the 24th and Laurie will fly out tomorrow. She has to be back at work, but promised to come out for a long weekend next month. Ron will go back to work August 1st. I can't look too far ahead without becoming engulfed with confusion and fear. I don't know what I'm going to do when life gets back to normal. Will there ever be "normal" without Joseph?

July 23

Sandy came by for a final visit today. She and Eva were at the funeral, but there wasn't much of an opportunity to talk. Sandy made a point of telling Ron and me what a good job we had done caring for Joseph. "In my six years with hospice, I've worked with many families, and I will always remember the love and caring that surrounded Joseph every minute of his life."

Sandy also left a booklet on the death of a child and information on the Infant Loss Support Group that hospice offers. Ron and I plan to attend their August meeting. I told Sandy that, when I felt stronger, I might want to be a volunteer with hospice. Ron and I thanked her for all the many ways she helped us in the past three weeks.

As soon as we have finished genetic counseling, Ron wants us to try for another baby. We both know a new baby will not replace Joseph. We just have so much love to give to a child. I'm not ready to think about it yet, but it helps to have some hope, to think about the possibility of having a baby. I have a lot of work to do on my fears. I want to believe that we can have a healthy baby. I want to have a baby that we will have here to love for a long time. I know, though, that the baby I want is Joseph.

When I began writing this journal life was very different. It seems like an eternity ago, and far away from this present emptiness. Laurie encourages me to continue writing, and I intend to. This seems like a safe place to put my questions and doubts, and to say how things are honestly, without editing it or protecting anyone. There is a purging, a relief that comes with it. I believe it will help me face the days ahead.

> *We find a place for what we lose. Although we know that after such a loss the acute stage of mourning will subside, we also know that we shall remain inconsolable and will never find a substitute. No matter what may fill the gap, even if it be filled completely, it nevertheless remains something else. And actually this is how it should be. It is the only way of perpetuating that love which we do not want to relinquish.*
>
> *—Letters of Sigmund Freud, 1961*

PEDIATRIC HOSPICE CARE
Care of Children Who Are Dying

Care of dying children, or pediatric hospice care, is one of the more important applications of hospice principles. Hospice pediatric services, like all hospice services, focus on the multidimensional needs of the child, and extend to the parents and family members who are grieving the impending death of the child. There are a number of elements involved in hospice care for children that differentiates it from hospice care of adults:

- *Demographics:* Mortality rates from childhood diseases are declining, and there are small numbers of children in need of hospice services.
- *Age:* There is a broad range of needs involved in care of children from birth to young adulthood. In addition to chronological age, developmental level and medical condition are powerful influences upon care.
- *Diagnosis:* Children die of terminal illnesses like cancer and also of a diverse set of chronic or terminal conditions, like Joseph's congenital anomalies, or cystic fibrosis. A broad range of staff knowledge and a diverse set of services are required.
- *Length of Hospice Care:* It is often more uncertain when a disease in a child is terminal, and when hospice care is appropriate. Late referrals make the length of stay in a hospice program of care typically short for a child.[1]

Care of Families

Hospice care for children offers some important benefits to parents and extended family members. The central focus, as it was in Joseph's care, is upon the quality of life and time spent together. There are also some unique qualities of families involved in caring for their child. When the child who is dying is young, the family is typically larger, including grandparents or siblings in addition to parents. Larger families generally represent greater availability of support, but can also mean more differences or conflicts. And, because parents always feel a sense of responsibility for young children, actual physical caregiving and participation in care is important. Dealing with the death of a child in any circumstances is an extremely painful and complicated task for all family members.

Hospice Caregivers

Hospice professionals and volunteers are highly skilled and trained in the care of adults who are dying. Care of children involves a particular set of needs that demands specific skills, knowledge, and approaches. Most hospices do not have sufficient populations of children to justify distinct programs. Rather, staff are recruited who have the specialized skills needed for work with children who are dying and their families. Because children have limited abilities to communicate, expert attention to pain and symptom control is required.

In general, pediatric hospice caregivers face greater challenges that require more sensitivity along with expert knowledge and skills. The role-related and emotional stresses involved in working with children who are dying can have a major impact.[2] Recruitment, careful selection, and support of staff providing care for children who are dying and their families are required of hospice programs.

Home Care and Inpatient Services

Although most of the care of children who are dying takes place in the home, inpatient settings may also be involved. For example, some neonatal intensive care units offer a family room and interdisciplinary hospice support for infants who will survive for only a brief time. Pediatric oncology centers that have been involved in the long-term care and treatment of a child with cancer often extend hospice services for a child who is dying. Because of their long-standing relationship with the child and the family, the pediatric oncology staff could be in a central and unique position to offer support. Care of young children with AIDS often requires periodic inpatient services. A range of services tailored to meet the unique needs of the child who is dying and of the family is optimal.

The Death of a Child

The death of a child can cause more severe suffering for family members than the death of an adult. Children represent our personal investment and legacy for the future. What Joseph's family grieved for over his death included all the unfulfilled potential of the relationship, all of the experiences that they would never have with him. The unique sorrows parents and family members experience surrounding a child's death include:

- Loss of the future
- Loss of the dreams attached to the child
- Loss of part of the self
- Failure of the parental role of protection
- Survivor's guilt (see chapter 3, p. 80)
- Reversal of the natural order of death
- Changes in family roles and functioning

While some of these concerns are present in all major losses, there is an intensification of the distress related to the death of a child. Death of a child during the first two years of life or during adolescence can present distinct problems related to separation. Joseph's parents had difficulty forming and letting go of the attachment at the same time. They were getting to know him, and also knew they would have to watch him die. During developmental transition times, when the child or adolescent is in the process of separating and differentiating from the parent, conflict and ambivalence can be high, complicating the grief process for parents whose children die. The inner emotional conflicts for parents in situations like these are sometimes great.

Bereavement Services

A key goal of caring for a child who is dying involves offering bereavement support to the family. Hospices are unique in the provision of bereavement care and services. The approach is truly a preventive one that includes contact with the family for a year following the child's death. The focus of offering bereavement support to the parents and any siblings involves the *general goals of all hospice bereavement services:*

- To provide family members with *information* about the normal grief process
- To provide grieving family members a *supportive opportunity* to review and reflect upon the experience of caring for their loved one and their loss experience
- To *assess and monitor* individual coping ability, risk and stress levels, and available support
- To *refer* and *encourage* family members to *access* and utilize existing support systems or to seek and create additional sources of support.[3]

The supportive resources that hospices themselves offer to bereaved parents may include support groups or grief courses for bereaved parents More recently, hospices have offered services to bereaved siblings such as play therapy, art therapy sessions, or "bereavement camps" for children, often held annually. In addition, many hospice programs work with teachers around ways to support grieving children in the school setting. Hospices may also refer to, or collaborate with, self-help groups like the Compassionate Friends.

An additional area of responsibility for hospice bereavement services involves having knowledge about appropriate mental health professionals to use as referral resources. Philosophically, hospices seek to fill gaps in community bereavement services and to coordinate and collaborate with existing services. Hospice programs are a part of the support equation available to families during the time of their great sorrow and need.

And can it be that in a world so full and busy, the loss of one weak creature makes a void in any heart, so wide and deep that nothing but the width and depth of vast eternity can fill it up!

— CHARLES DICKENS
Dombey and Son

Chapter Five

THE COMMITMENT
Facing the End of Life His Own Way

Walter Adams sat in his green recliner, his back to the sun-filled window, dozing and thinking. He knew this cancer was gnawing away inside him, out of control. At least there had been the six-year reprieve. He'd never considered facing the end of his life, even at 82. He supposed that everyone wants more time, assumes more time, expects more time. It wasn't so much the fact of dying. He just hoped that he'd be here longer, to enjoy more, discover more.

If there was anything Walter appreciated in life it was learning. Though he had never gone beyond his bachelor's degree, his life's work was education. Maybe that's what made him such a well-regarded teacher. He loved to explore and ask questions. Socrates was right. Asking questions is the secret to learning.

Since the recurrence of his colon cancer, Walter seemed to be in the grip of endless questions. There was a disquieting quality to this time. Not that he'd changed any of his beliefs. He was just thinking about them more, examining them carefully.

The previous February he'd gone for his scheduled visit to the gastroenterologist. Walter didn't like Dr. Packard's closed, aloof manner. When he told Walter about the recurrence, he reported the bad news briefly, factually, and left no room for discussion. He was literally passing him off to the care of Dr. Taylor, an oncologist. Because of the spread of the cancer, he was not recommending additional surgery. He ended by saying, "And, well, at your age, there are fewer considerations." Walter wanted to strike back and say, "What do you know about who I am, and how I live at my age? I still walk a mile or two several times a week. I participate in the current affairs discussion groups at the civic center, and I volunteer two days a week at the junior high school. And then there's Carol. We've been married for fifty-six years. We still travel together, play bridge, take wildflower hikes, and spend evenings rich with music, food, and friends. Does all that have to end?"

Tears often veiled Carol's eyes now. It was lonelier because Walter didn't say much. He sat in his recliner and thought a lot more, for hours each day. She could see him rolling over the progression of questions and arguments he was raising in his mind. They were the questions he always considered when things were difficult. When Carol asked him what he was thinking about, he thinly replied, "I'm just sorting things through." It was his way of saying that there would be no discussion.

Carol told Walter that she needed to sort things out as well. "We could do some of the considering together. I need to talk with you." Walter would say, "I can't now," and walk away. Carol thought this was more than his everyday stubbornness. He had pulled so much more into himself and was further away from her than she ever remembered.

In the weeks that followed, there were several medications that the oncologist tried on Walter. Each one left him retching or doubled over with diarrhea. For many years, Walter and Carol had discussed not having excessive treatments or procedures. While he was hoping the new medication would bring him some response or a reprieve, he wasn't willing to feel this bad. The side effects were too much for him. On a visit in early April to Dr. Taylor's oncology office, the nurse suggested a referral to hospice. Walter rankled at the idea, and Carol felt it was premature. Their friend Valerie had worked as a hospice volunteer for a number of years. Walter and Carol decided they would talk with her about the right time to involve hospice.

For more than a decade, Walter and Carol had participated in end-of-life decision-making discussions at their church and at the senior club in town. They each had a current will, a durable power of attorney, and specific advance directives. After Walter's initial cancer diagnosis, they had both spoken with their internist, Dr. Bannock, about their desires to avoid unnecessary and invasive treatment. They were both members in good standing of the Hemlock Society, a grassroots organization dedicated to advancing the individual right to end-of-life choices, including assisted suicide. Carol wanted to talk with Walter about his wishes now, but she hesitated to bring it up. The last thing she wanted to do was to make Walter feel that she was wanting to hurry his departure. It was one thing to talk about the right to die when it was an abstract issue, and quite another thing to consider it when the threat of death was hovering close.

The most Walter would say was that it was "miserable to feel this way." It was wrenching for Carol to watch him experience such demeaning symptoms. "It's not a way to live" he told Valerie one day when she visited. And that was all he said. Carol wanted to hear more about hospice and the services they offered, but she knew Walter wouldn't consider it. She wondered if he would ever really feel ready for hospice.

Two weeks later, Walter was feeling more pain and having growing gastrointestinal distress each day. Carol felt like she was floundering with all the symptoms. "I don't know what to do to make him more comfortable. When I called Dr. Taylor, the oncologist, he suggested we contact the local hospice. He said, 'they're the pain control experts.'"

When Valerie visited that afternoon, she knew that Carol hoped she could convince Walter to agree to hospice services. Valerie decided to focus their conversation on just a few of the services that hospice would offer. She didn't want Walter to feel pushed or defensive. "I have seen the hospice team do an excellent job of managing pain and physical symptoms. From medications and diet to everyday home remedies, they are able to help people feel more comfortable. There are two other things you might want to consider, Walter. First, it seems to me that Carol's telling you that she could use some help, and I know that you care about her and want her to be okay. Second, I know how careful you have both been with money and how much you appreciate a good deal."

All three of them smiled and Walter let a little chuckle out. "It's our Depression legacy, I guess."

"One of the best things about hospice is that the Medicare benefit will cover most of your expenses. And that includes paying for the majority of medication expenses, too," Valerie concluded.

Walter was quiet for a few moments. "I didn't know that. That's an important help. I remember when Carol was so sick with septic pneumonia last fall, after she was discharged from the hospital we had to pay for the medications, and the antibiotics cost so much. I still feel that I'm not ready for hospice, though."

"Well, in the best of all worlds, if you have a remission, you can be discharged from hospice. So, you really have nothing to lose."

"Well, I suppose if you think it's a good idea—and, I know Carol wants help."

"If you'd like, I'll call Donna, the patient-care coordinator at hospice, and see about getting you a great nurse. I think you both will appreciate the special attention and support that hospice offers."

When Valerie phoned hospice to request services for Walter and Carol, she explained Walter's hesitations to Donna, the patient-care coordinator. Donna responded with a promise to let the assigned nurse know that a gentle, low-key approach with Walter would be important.

The next day, Barbara, the hospice nurse, phoned and set the appointment for the initial assessment at 4 P.M. that afternoon. Barbara was in her early fifties and had been working with hospice almost nine years. She had learned to proceed carefully with families on the first visit. Even though people had agreed to hospice care, that didn't mean that they welcomed the idea of hospice and the end of life. From the patient-care coordinator's comments, Barbara knew that the Adamses were struggling with how briskly things were advancing.

Once Walter made a decision, he stood with it. So when Barbara arrived he was friendly and interested. A part of him still didn't believe that he could be so ill. Carol was both anxious and relieved to have hospice involved. She knew the situation was more than she could cope with, and yet she was determined to handle things. She and Walter had made an agreement long ago that neither of them would put the other in a nursing home. Now, with the help of hospice, she intended to keep that promise.

Dorothy, the hospice social worker, accompanied Barbara on the first visit. Together they offered information about the services, discussed the difficulties Walter and Carol were experiencing, and inquired about the kinds of supportive services they would find helpful. After looking over brochures and booklets, Walter and Carol signed the various admission papers. Barbara promised to contact Dr. Taylor to sort out the medications that would work with Walter's symptoms. She also spoke with Carol about diet and food preparation. Both Walter and Carol felt that the visit had gone well.

After several attempts with different pain medications, the one that worked best for Walter was an analgesic patch that he wore for forty-eight to seventy-two hours and then changed. It helped ease the spasms and pain, and Walter appreciated not having to take more pills. He still awakened two or three times each night to go to the bathroom, but he didn't need to get Carol up, and usually he could get back to sleep.

Walter's advancing illness had brought about major changes in Carol's activities. Before his recurrence, she hiked once or twice a week with the local senior's club and she was on the board of two community organizations. When Walter had become ill, she had resigned from one board and decided to take a leave from her involvement with the low-income clinic she had helped found fifteen years before. If Walter felt more stable, Carol would occasionally take a long walk.

In the last week, Barbara had brought some liquid protein supplements and they helped both Walter and Carol feel less worried about keeping his strength up. Now he ate the things he wanted and often requested something he was in the mood for. He even asked for hot dogs one day, and Carol happily prepared them. Carol felt good when he asked for a certain food and then was actually able to enjoy it. Lately that was happening about half the time.

During the first two weeks that hospice began caring for Walter and Carol, they were visited by the hospice chaplain, Don Ellis. Walter was an agnostic and believed that death was the absolute end. When the hospice chaplain visited, they began discussing beliefs about death and afterlife. Don asked Walter how his faith was helping him during his illness. "I don't think of faith in those terms. My beliefs have always involved a sense of exploration of important life issues and a sense of social consciousness. As far as dying goes, the only way I know that we live on is in the hearts and minds of the people we have loved and influenced. I can't bring myself to see death as anything but final. I've had these beliefs for most of my life, and Carol shares them as well."

Don listened carefully and then asked Walter, "How do your beliefs make this time of your life easier?"

Walter pondered for a moment. "I'm not sure. I know that I do want to talk about some of these issues at times. I'm enjoying our conversation, and I've had similar ones with friends. It seems like a difficult time to change beliefs, when you're facing the end of your life. It probably would be more comforting to see things differently. After all these years these beliefs are just a part of me, of how I see the world and life. I don't know how I can approach all this any differently now."

Don responded, "Well, I think that it's important to hold

to our beliefs, even when it's difficult to do that. It seems to me that beliefs are like the boat we sail in through our life. I admire the integrity you show when you talk about how you see the end of life, and you're right, it might be easier now if you thought that life went on in some fashion. Sometimes, though, when we are in difficult circumstances, we reexamine our beliefs and question whether they still fit for us, given what we know now. It seems like you have done that, and the answer is that these are your beliefs, even in this difficult time."

For a few minutes the two men were silent, then Walter asked Don, "What do you think of a person taking his life before death takes him?"

Don looked at Walter and wondered how personal the question was. "Well, I have mixed feelings. It's not an easy question. In my twenty-three years as a chaplain, I've seen people in a wide range of painful times. And, I'm not just talking about physical pain. The nurses and doctors can handle that well. It's more the other kinds of pain—the losing control, the helplessness, the hard work of separating and leave-taking, or of wanting to protect the people we love from what we see as the "burdens" of caregiving. Those things seem to be what I've heard as people struggle with the end of life. What do you think about ending your own life, Walter?" Don asked.

"Both Carol and I have been members of the Hemlock Society for years, and we have an agreement about neither of us putting the other in a nursing home. I've been so independent all my life, I dread the thought of becoming weaker and not able to care for myself. And colon cancer is not a very dignified disease. I suppose that if my diarrhea gets worse, or if there's more tumor growth, I'll be wearing a diaper. That's a terrible thought for me, and I honestly don't know if Carol can handle this. She gets flustered pretty easily and is quite fragile herself. I've always been the one to carry a major portion of the load around here. I think if things got much worse, I would consider ending my life."

"It's always a human option to take one's own life," Don offered. "It seems like we need the reassurance of knowing that we could leave if things get too difficult. That knowledge in itself can be sustaining. Walter, are there any reasons *not* to end your life prematurely?"

"Of course there are. Carol and I would talk about it, and I assume she would need to help me if I made that decision. She would have a difficult time with it when faced with the reality though. I know it would be very painful for her to let me go. And our daughter, Kim, would likely be very upset. She may understand, but she would have wanted a chance to know, or to be here. I imagine if I make the decision to end my life, I won't be telling many people. I would probably just tell Carol."

Don considered the dilemma Walter was facing. "I honestly don't know that I would feel any differently if I were in your position, Walter. I can only tell you what I have seen in the families that I've worked with across the years. You are right, it would be difficult for Carol and Kim. Family members seem to feel a sense of failure and of greater abandonment. Even if that isn't the reality, they emotionally feel a great conflict. Usually family members focus on the question, 'Is there something else that I could have done, or some other way that I could have helped?' So there is more of a sense of helplessness for the family.

"And, there's another piece," Don continued. "One of the good things that happens when family members care for someone they love is that there are some unique opportunities for closeness and loving. That seems to matter a great deal to the people I've known. As I heard you say earlier, Walter, we never have enough time with the people we love. We are always left wishing we had more. So, I don't have any easy answer. Working with hospice has taught me that there are other things that we can focus on before we talk about suicide. Things like being comfortable, and quality of life, and time with people we love. If those things are happening, then even when other things are rough, we can live through them to the natural conclusion and suicide isn't an issue anymore. Or, if the feeling of not being able to face what lies ahead comes up, we choose to hang in there a bit longer, and then it passes."

"Well, I'm not contemplating it for today or tomorrow. It is certainly something I do consider and choose to keep open as a possibility." Walter smiled at Don. "I appreciate your not preaching at me, or trying to save my immortal soul today."

Don smiled back. "And I'm grateful that you trusted me enough to talk about all this with me. You're a good man, Walter, a man who stands by his principles. I respect and admire that. Would it be okay if I visited you again in a week or so?"

Walter agreed. "I'd like that. I've enjoyed our conversation."

During the next two weeks, Walter's weakness sank deeper into his being. "I'm tired of being tired," he told Carol. "It's even difficult to walk across the room some of the time. And I'm tired of the cycles of diarrhea and constipation."

Walter was very worried about developing a bowel obstruction. He informed Barbara, the hospice nurse, "If I have to choose between diarrhea and constipation, I choose diarrhea." Barbara agreed that she would try to adjust the medications and diet recommendations so that constipation was not a problem for Walter. Walter responded, "It seems like we're just putting out brushfires here. Soon there will be another to contend with."

"It's been a rough few days for you, Walter. Is there anything else bothering you besides feeling weak and the constipation?" Barbara asked.

"I think I'm just tired of being sick, of not being able to do things. Mostly, I'm just more irritable today. I didn't sleep well last night. I was up so many times and felt so bloated.

Carol was sound asleep, and even though I was so uncomfortable, I didn't want to wake her. I'm worried about what we will do as time goes on."

Barbara was solid in her offer of reassurance. "It seems important that you let Carol know when you need her during the night. And, if things are too difficult for her, we can get some respite care in when you both need it. There are five days and nights of respite care available to you through hospice. If you would like to hire additional help, we can give you a list of people we recommend. It's not helpful for you to feel alone when you are feeling sick like last night, Walter. When Carol gets back from the store, would it be all right with you if we talked with her about this?"

"I suppose so," Walter agreed. "I just don't want to add to her worries even more."

"Of course she's worried. She loves you and this is hard for her, too. What seems to work best, though, is when you both let each other know what's important. Not knowing is harder, don't you think?"

Walter resolved the conversation, "I guess it's time we talked a bit more about what we're going to need to get through this."

Three days later, Walter had an episode of acute abdominal pain along with rectal bleeding. It was just before 11 P.M. when Carol phoned the hospice nurse on call and she arrived within twenty minutes. Because Walter was losing a significant amount of blood and experiencing acute pain, the hospice nurse called Dr. Taylor's office. He directed them to meet him at the hospital emergency room. After examining Walter, Dr. Taylor admitted him to the hospice inpatient unit at the hospital for observation until the bleeding stopped and his pain was brought under control.

Carol was frightened. "I don't think I can handle this. I never thought it would be this difficult. I'm not sure how much more I can take." The hospice social worker, Dorothy, listened as Carol talked and cried.

"Walter has a good chance of stabilizing. You can use the

time while he's on the unit to rest and gather up your energy again. I'll see you tomorrow and we can talk more about what will help you and Walter most now." Carol nodded and agreed that it would help just to be able to rest a bit.

The following day, Walter's bleeding stopped. When Carol came in to see him, she went to see Dorothy first. Together they talked about what additional services would be needed when Walter returned home. Because Walter was increasingly weak, a nursing assistant would now come in three times a week to help with personal care. Dorothy and Carol then went in and talked with Walter about plans for respite care during the night so that Carol could sleep. Carol was worried about the expense of additional respite care, but they decided to try it for a week. Walter reassured Carol that there would be enough money to cover the respite costs. According to Dorothy, the local hospice had received a grant to fund a pilot project of coordinating and training a group of lay personal-care providers, so the costs would be less than usual for additional respite care.

After they left Walter's room, Dorothy asked Carol what else might be helpful for her. Carol responded, "I just can't believe this is happening. I know there's nothing I can do to stop Walter's illness. Caring for him is more difficult than I imagined. It seems like we have always been together. It scares me when he talks about ending his life. I'm just not ready to have him go yet. I don't know what I would do if he asked me to help him."

"Maybe you need to let him know the things you've just told me," Dorothy offered. "Walter's a very reasonable and caring man. If he knows how you feel, that would matter to him. Does your daughter, Kim, have any plans to visit soon? I know you've told me how close she is to Walter, and a visit from her might help you both. We just can't say exactly how much time Walter has, but it doesn't look like it will be more than a month or two. If she wants to see him when he still has energy and can really enjoy her visit, she may want to come soon."

"She's been wanting to come, and waiting for me to tell her when it is right. Maybe this is the time. I could use her help now as well," Carol acknowledged.

Walter was discharged from the hospice inpatient unit two days later. Kim arrived the following Saturday to stay with her parents for five days. Carol was relieved and grateful for Kim's help with Walter's care and with household tasks. While they both avoided discussing serious matters, Walter and Kim enjoyed their usual conversations and warm displays of affection. "We didn't know how much we needed to see you, Kim. It's made such a difference for both of us to have you here," Walter acknowledged. Barbara, the hospice nurse, commented both to the Adamses during her regular visit and at the hospice interdisciplinary team meeting that week that the entire family had been buoyed by Kim's visit. "The difference in the way they're dealing with things is remarkable."

As the days passed, Walter and Carol were able to sustain their calm and determined manners. When Walter had a difficult day Carol was able to respond to his needs with less anxiety. "I need to do this for Walter," she reasoned. "That's just how it is. He certainly has taken care of me when I've been ill. That may have been my biggest worry: who would care for me. When Kim was here I felt sure that she would be there when I needed her. That made a big difference. And the respite help at night has been good. I'm still up with Walter a few nights a week, but I'm getting more sleep now so I feel more able to cope with everything."

Don, the hospice chaplain, called and came by for a second visit with Walter that week. "I hear you've had some rough days since we last visited, Walter."

Walter agreed. "A couple of weeks ago I didn't think I'd make it through the night. We might not have had this second conversation we agreed upon. Thank goodness things are a bit easier now. Still, I'm losing ground every day. It's hard to walk across the room to get to my recliner some days. We will probably need to make this visit a shorter one. I don't last very long these days. It seems that I'm sleeping on and off a lot during the day."

"Just let me know when you're feeling tired, Walter, and I'll leave. I appreciate your seeing me today. Tell me how things have been with you lately," Don inquired.

Thinking for a moment, Walter began, "Well, things certainly haven't been easy. It is very troublesome for me to lose my physical capabilities. I guess I would say that we seem to be handling things pretty well now, though. We reached a turning point when I had the bleeding episode and went to the hospice inpatient unit. After that, Kim, our daughter, who lives in D.C., was here for almost a week. That helped us both out a lot. Carol seems to be doing better with the help at night, too. All in all, things seem to be going as well as we could expect. This is just not much of a way to live."

"I'm glad that things have evened out for you and Carol. When you say that this is not much of a way to live, tell me more about what that means for you, Walter. Where are you with the early leave-taking pact that you and Carol have?"

"Honestly, I haven't thought about that decision as much lately," Walter admitted. "I'm not sure why. It's not that I like the spot I'm in. And I know it's only going to get worse. Right now, though, things seem to be tolerable, and Carol and I have some good moments. She seems to be stronger now. I haven't closed out the possibility that I may choose a hasty exit; I just don't seem to feel much inclination in that direction now. I'm looking forward to Kim coming back in the next month or so, and that will be good."

Don was sitting in a chair at a right angle to Walter's green recliner. "It's good to hear that things are smoother for you for now, Walter. Have you thought about how you might feel when you become more ill or weak?"

Walter looked out the large picture window framing the bright branches of June trees. "I've been trying not to look too far ahead. I find I'm better off just dealing with the things at hand. As I said before, I'm not willing to close out any of my options. Right now, though, things seem manageable," Walter concluded.

Don nodded. "They do, and I'm glad. Have you thought about what seems to offer you the most comfort now, Walter?"

"It's a combination of things, I guess. It helps that Carol and I seem to be doing well, and I look forward to seeing Kim again. The stronger patches have helped the pain and spasms and that makes all the difference in my outlook. All the attention from the hospice people doesn't hurt either. I especially like our nurse, Barbara. She's a gem."

Don smiled and agreed. "People do seem to make a difference, don't they? Maybe that's the formula that will work best for you, Walter. Relationships give our lives meaning, and you certainly have many people who think well of you. I can see how important it is for you to have people close by at this time."

"I might not have put it that way, but it's true. I can see that Carol feels less alone now, and I'm appreciating the people that I see. My energy's gone, though, Don. I'm afraid you'll have to excuse me, but I need to rest again now." After saying good-bye to both Walter and Carol, Don left the Adams home feeling much less concerned than he had on his last visit.

During the next week Walter experienced growing weakness and restlessness. When Kim heard the distress in her mother's voice, she called Valerie and asked whether she thought that it was time for her to come out again. Carol had not asked Kim to come when she had called earlier that evening. "My mother told me that the hospice nurse said that Dad might only last another week or two. I'm not sure whether I should come out now."

Valerie listened and responded, "When I saw your dad earlier today, your mom said that he is no longer able to eat much. He occasionally takes a little liquid protein supplement. And he's sleeping a lot now. I think that your mother would welcome your coming, and be relieved. How would it be for you to see your father this ill?"

"I think I could handle it. I don't want to wait until after he dies. I want to be there for both of them. So I guess that I have made my decision."

Three days later, Kim arrived. She helped her mother with household chores as well as with her father's care. They had an aide there every night as Walter's restlessness increased. Dr. Taylor added a new medication and Walter was more peaceful now. He slept a great deal and got up only to use the bedside commode. Kim was pleased to see the tenderness and loving care her mother was giving her father. She knew how tired her mother was, and what little sleep she was getting. "It seems like this has been going on for a long time. I'm so glad you're here," Carol told Kim. "I really needed you, and I know your dad does, too."

Two days later, Walter told Kim he wanted to sit in his recliner. That afternoon, Kim and the aide got Walter up to sit in his favorite chair, which they had moved into the bedroom. When he was settled in, Carol pulled up a chair and sat beside him. When she reached over to offer him some water, he touched her face and kissed her cheek.

Later, Kim sat near her father and spoke to him, telling him how much she loved him. "I know that you can't talk, Dad, but I know that you can hear me. I want to tell you how much I love having you for a dad. We have always been pals, doing things together. You even built me that tree house. And you were always such a good teacher, so encouraging and supportive of me and of the things that I wanted to pursue."

Hesitantly, Kim continued, "Now I want to talk to you about some of the things that I've read about in recent years, things that I believe. It all started when my friend Sally died so suddenly from a brain aneurysm. I don't think that our lives end here. I believe that life continues on, though I'm not sure exactly how. I do believe that we will be together again someday, and that belief gives me great comfort. In some ways, it makes it possible to let you go. I'm not sure where you are with your beliefs now, Dad, but I hope that in some corner of your mind or heart you will keep open the possibility of some continuity of life. That's a gift you could give yourself and me. I want so much for you to be at peace now." After a brief moment, Walter opened his eyes, looked at Kim, and squeezed her hand gently. That evening, after Walter was back in bed, he became unresponsive, lapsing into a coma-like state.

Two days later, Walter died in his sleep. At about 7 P.M. his slow breathing just stopped. Carol phoned the hospice nurse, who arrived a half hour later. Meanwhile, Valerie and her husband, Larry, came in response to Carol's call, giving them news of Walter's death. They stayed with the family as they talked and said good-byes to Walter.

When the memorial service was held the following Tuesday, over two hundred friends attended. Kim gave a moving reminiscence about her father, and numerous friends spoke of Walter's great wit, warmth, and intelligence. Kim stayed on for the rest of the week, with a promise to visit her mother again in six weeks.

Five days later, Carol received a visit from Barbara, the hospice nurse. Barbara told Carol what an impressive job she had done caring for Walter, especially in light of his many difficult symptoms. Gratefully, Carol acknowledged that she hadn't always been sure that she could do it. "The respite care and aides made all the difference in my being able to care for him here at home, where he wanted to be. And Kim's help at the end was so important. I'm just so pleased that we could do it for Walter."

Don, the hospice chaplain, phoned Carol and asked if he could come by. His visit came exactly four weeks after Walter's death. After inquiring about how Carol was coping, Don shared some of the conversations that he had had with Walter. "He loved you very much. So much that he even considered ending his life to spare you the hardship of caring for him."

"I know," Carol admitted. "We just reached a point when it was no longer a consideration. He just needed to have an out in case he wanted it. Once the pain and discomfort eased, he was able to deal with things better. I was, too. The time in the inpatient hospice unit made a big difference for both of us. After that, things seemed to fall into place better for us. It wasn't easy, and I couldn't have done it without hospice. But I'm awfully glad that I was able to care for Walter. He was a rare man, a gentle man with a love of life and people. I'm very lucky to have shared fifty-six years with him. I miss him dearly. I know that I'll be missing him all the rest of my days."

It is necessary; therefore, it is possible.

—G. A. BORGHESE

Unique Concerns of the Elderly

Elderly couples face a complicated set of problems in dealing with their spouse's imminent death. Separating from a person we love is one of the greatest costs of an intimate relationship. The generation who lived as couples through the Depression and a world war, raised children together, and now face diminishment and death are a rare group in our culture today. Ironically, reliance upon another person has been the topic of debate and dispute in recent years. From feminist perspectives on autonomy in relationships to the fear of "codependency" and the advent of serial monogamy, the character and commitments of relationships have changed.

Carol and Walter Adams shared an unusual closeness, with their marriage forming the foundation that encouraged other involvements. Many aspects of their story reflect the coping and health of their generation. While their communication may not have always been open, their approach to problems was typically a jointly shared process, one that included their partner.

Coping in Extreme Moments

Individuals and families facing the end of life struggle with a myriad of problems and distressing emotions. Both Walter and Carol were forced to deal with feelings of frustration, anxiety, hopelessness, and a time perspective where the walls seemed to be closing in on them. They each doubted their individual abilities to handle their situation. Because of their age and circumstances, both Walter and Carol felt extremely vulnerable. Feelings of despair can be at the core of vulnerability. Vulnerability erodes self-confidence and morale, while effective coping strengthens them. Effective coping and problem-solving activities counterbalance vulnerability and distress, and yet, in times of greatest vulnerability and distress, coping abilities typically and naturally recede.[1]

Coping is the term used to denote all of the mechanisms utilized by an individual to meet a significant threat to his or her stability. Coping behaviors involve adaptation and enable effective functioning.[2] Beyond survival, reaching a personally defined quality of life requires that we cope with the problems that present themselves in our lives. The ability to cope well demands that we recognize the gap between what we want and what can be expected, or what is presently possible. In times of vulnerability, coping becomes a necessary, incessant, and enduring process.

The goal of all coping efforts is to regain a sense of hope and direction that can regenerate quality of life. Across time, we learn what works and what doesn't work for us in various situations of our lives. Observers have long seen that people differ widely in their capacities and abilities to face problems, cope, and maintain diminished levels of vulnerability.

There is no magic formula for coping that would be useful for all families facing the terminal phases of an illness.

Coping strategies are more like a bag of tricks that we pull from as needed. Positive coping requires that we employ more than one strategy, and that the problem be addressed directly. Avoidance and denial limit our abilities to deal with the problems at hand. If there is a continuum of coping and well-being, good coping and the potential for well-being are on the attention end of the continuum, while distress and poor coping are on the avoidance pole of the continuum.[3]

Optimism is always highly correlated with good coping and also with well-being. In addition, people who cope well tend to be resourceful, accepting available support as well as looking to their own inner resources. A problem-solving approach that involves awareness and acceptance, considers alternatives, and focuses on solutions is important.

At the outset, Walter and Carol had difficulties coping with their changed life situation. Both crumpled under the initial blow of Walter's cancer recurrence and rapid decline. The problems that they faced seemed overwhelming, and they avoided dealing with them together, or with the help of many outside resources. Eventually, they were able to face their circumstances and access and utilize support in adaptive ways.

When Walter experienced his physical crisis and was admitted to the hospice inpatient unit, some major coping was required of both Walter and Carol. They were no longer able to continue avoiding their realities. The suggestions and plans generated with the hospice staff helped Walter and Carol feel more capable upon his return home, and experience a greater sense of control.

Significant survival, or an acceptable quality of life, requires options, respect, reasonable security, and a sense of living up to the potential or within the scope of what is esteemed.

—AVERY WEISMAN[4]

The Role of Faith

Faith plays a central role in the constellation of coping responses to a life-threatening illness or death of a loved one. Beliefs are tools that can enable survival. They are the structure or a house that we build for our lives so that we can live inside them. Holding personal beliefs, or having faith, can focus our energies and minimize our fears. Faith can also have a balancing effect, helping people rediscover hope and peacefulness.

A life-threatening illness or death of a loved one forces us to continue to reframe what we believe in, and what we pray for. Early on, the person diagnosed with a life-threatening illness and family members may pray and hope for a cure. By believing that cure or remission is possible, we demonstrate a measure of trust in life, as well as in God.

Difficult times test our faith. Because of the influence of the cause-and-effect nature of puritan-type thinking, we feel punished when we experience painful realities. It is almost an instinctive response to examine ways in which we could have "brought on" or caused the illness or death. Out of our powerlessness, we look for a reason why painful experiences happen; then, if there is a predictable cause, we try to find comfort in the belief that there is a pattern and order to our universe. Somehow, believing that there is a reason or cause for suffering can give us a feeling of safety.

Numerous spiritual writers and thinkers discuss the sustaining nature of faith during difficult times. In discussing the fact that most Jews upheld their faith during the Holocaust, Burkle comments, "They continued to believe in God whether or not they could find good reasons for doing so."[5]

A Sustaining Influence

One of the major difficulties surrounding a life-threatening illness is that it shrinks our world to a locus of concern about physical changes and symptoms. In other ways, a life-threatening illness or loss of a loved one sharply clarifies our values and helps us rediscover and attend to those things that are most important in our lives. Perhaps the greatest comfort of faith lies in our sense of a personal relationship with God.

Faith has the powerful ability to strengthen us in ordinary and painful times of our lives. It allows us to transcend our concerns and focus on the caring or knowing presence of a god figure. The comfort that faith can offer to people who believe is immense.

The spiritual matters of faith and prayer change and grow as the experience of the illness and dying process evolves. Sometimes faith is initially wrapped around the hope for a cure, and then unfolds into less specific hopes and prayers. Across time, faith can be a powerful personal resource.

> *It isn't enough to believe in something; you have to have the stamina to meet obstacles and overcome them, to struggle."*
>
> —GOLDA MEIR

Prayer

Beliefs can lead to a call for help in troubled times. For some, prayer becomes a petition or cry for intercession on our behalf, or for someone we love. There is a progression of praying that unfolds, where first we are hoping for a cure, then for a remission, for more time, fewer symptoms, the chance to experience some special event or accomplishment, and finally for good, peaceful moments at the end of our life. Many people also hope for continuity of life after death.

Unlike bargaining with our fate, prayer is often the expression of or a petition for the fulfillment of our hopes and wishes. If we invest in the possibility that our fate may brighten, we invest in the present, with some anticipation of the future.

For some, prayer is the act of seeking help from an omnipotent god. Thomas Merton, the contemplative Catholic theologian, offered a major insight into the practice in defining prayer as paying attention.[6] When we live in the present, we heighten our awareness and can discover things that connect us to life, things to be grateful for. Brother David Steindl-Rast believes that being alive means having a sense of gratefulness.[7] If we are paying attention, there is the potential to discover a number of things to feel grateful for, even in the most painful times of life.

Spiritual Needs

There is a difference between religious and spiritual concerns. Religious concerns are typically the focus of a specific faith congregation or community, and are attached to a generally agreed-upon set of doctrines. Spiritual needs are more global and go beyond particular religious beliefs to the consideration of personal beliefs and meanings.

Hospice's approach to care of the dying recognizes the importance of addressing the full spectrum of human needs. Spiritual needs are perhaps the ones that are most difficult to define, and the most personal. According to National Hospice Organization Standards, hospices initially and on an ongoing basis assess the spiritual needs of the person who is dying and of the family members. This assessment documents the historical and current religious affiliation of the dying person, and focuses on the nature and scope of the person's spiritual concerns and needs. These needs include:

- Reexamining beliefs
- Exploring beliefs about an afterlife
- Reconciling life choices
- Exploring one's lifetime contribution
- Examining loving relationships
- Discovering meaning

All of these spiritual concerns involve reflection and exploration. Some people do that examination in a meditative, solitary way, and do not speak of it with others. In themselves, the illness and dying process offer opportunities for understanding and healing that may never be shared with another person. Family members go through similar exploration processes, both during their loved one's illness and dying and during the time of bereavement.

Discovering Meaning

The discovery of meaning is a large and vague concept. Frankl sheds light on the quest for meaning by offering three ways to find meaning: (1) doing a deed; (2) experiencing a value; and (3) through suffering.[8] According to Frankl's understanding, experiencing a value includes experiencing someone through love. Frankl's original understanding grew out of his concentration camp experiences and his writings were rooted in day-to-day encounters with tragedy and death. Applying these sources of meaning to individuals and families facing death and to hospice care is valuable. Facing death as well as making the sacrifices involved in caregiving offer innumerable opportunities for discovering meaning. When all else falls away, the personal meaning we attribute to our lives is perhaps the most essential and valuable part of our individual humanness.

The Spiritual Strength of Relationships

In her revealing, personal introduction to *A Rumor of Angels*,[9] Alice Walker writes about her childhood closeness and reliance upon her older sister, Ruth. Walker talks about the transition from having Ruth beside her during difficult times in their childhood to their separation and the tight encirclement of grief she felt in her sister's absence. Walker tells of eventually developing a larger, more universal and sustaining spiritual experience. She extends her personal image of wanting to offer comfort for the readers by wishing her words could be for them what holding her sister's hand was like for her. In the strange terrain of grief, sorrow, and separation, caring human closeness is essential and offers spiritual strength. Again, the image of presence and journeying together resurfaces, this time in embarking upon spiritual territories that remain not only uncharted, but as mysterious as they are personal.

> *With this faith we will hew out of the mountain of despair the stone of hope.*
>
> —MARTIN LUTHER KING, JR.

Life-Threatening Illness

Separation, loss, and grief all interfere with our attachments, not just to the person(s) we love, but also to life itself. It is almost impossible to imagine our own non-being, or that of someone we love. We project our present circumstances into the future and assume that they will continue on. Impending death and the anticipatory grief that accompanies it shatter our assumptions and create a sense of unreality. The personal and private pain associated with anticipated death can trigger not just feelings of loss of control, but also existential despair. Irvin Yalom, noted professor of psychiatry at Stanford University School of Medicine, defines existential conflicts as those that flow from an individual's confrontation with the givens of existence, like death and grief.[10]

There is considerable discussion in Western cultures surrounding end-of-life concerns. Cultural values around autonomy and individual rights clash with dependency concerns and moral and religious questions. On the spectrum of decision-making related to life-threatening illness, assisted suicide and euthanasia represent the extreme pole of determination on the choice continuum. All points on the decision-making continuum involve communication as well as the exploration of values.

Communication and Advanced Decision-Making

Hospice programs across the country have encouraged families using their services to complete advance directives, living wills, do-not-resuscitate orders, and a durable power of attorney. These instruments promote discussion among family members as well as between the person who is ill with a life-threatening disease and the physician. Typically, there is inadequate communication between the person who is ill in a life-threatening circumstance and the physician about end-of-life care and wishes regarding treatment.[11] While there is often a sea of ambiguity churning in these dramatic situations, the lack of clear communication clouds the waters further.

Effective communication and information-sharing between physicians and those in life-threatening circumstances is crucial to sound decision-making. Hospice is often not presented or seen as an alternative in those situations when there are no longer any reasonable or effective curatives remaining. Families in the crisis of terminal or life-threatening illnesses are generally not assertive consumers

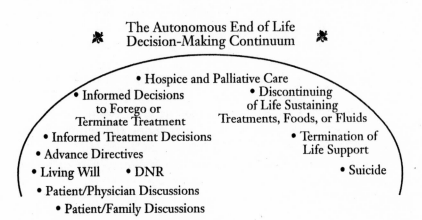

The Autonomous End of Life
Decision-Making Continuum

- Hospice and Palliative Care
- Informed Decisions to Forego or Terminate Treatment
- Discontinuing of Life Sustaining Treatments, Foods, or Fluids
- Informed Treatment Decisions
- Advance Directives
- Termination of Life Support
- Living Will
- DNR
- Suicide
- Patient/Physician Discussions
- Patient/Family Discussions

and are often not made aware of the choice of hospice care. When there is literally "nothing more to be done" in the realm of curative treatment, hospice can be presented as the option that offers a new "something to be done." Palliative care or symptom-focused comfort care can make a vital qualitative difference in the final months and weeks of life.

Hospice and the Decision-Making Continuum

Hospice programs, through their collective voice in the National Hospice Organization, have identified key issues in regard to the hospice approach to end-of-life care. These points not only define hospice values, they are also part of the organization's official position opposing assisted suicide and euthanasia:[12]

1. Every American deserves the option of the comprehensive symptom management and supportive care that hospice represents.
2. Hospice neither hastens nor postpones death.
3. Hospice effectively addresses the fears of painful suffering, abandonment, and loss of control.
4. Symptoms can be controlled and physical suffering can be alleviated.
5. Adequate symptom management is *not* euthanasia.
6. Depression is an underrecognized problem in terminal illness.
7. Autonomy rights of hospice patients are fully respected.
8. Financial devastation is currently part of the suffering of too many patients with life-limiting illness.
9. Assisted suicide or euthanasia, if legalized, would not solve the problems of caring for the terminally ill and might, indeed, distract from the effort.
10. Dying is not undignified. It is simply part of being human.

11. Dying is frequently a rich and meaningful process for individuals and their families.

Walter and Carol Adams' experience speaks loudly to many of these key issues. Based upon fears or misguided wishes to protect loved ones, the consideration of assisted suicide is never a clear-cut or simple concern. In fact, the ability to take one's own life is woven into the human condition. All of us have had moments when we questioned whether we were able or willing to continue on with our lives. For the vast majority, that feeling passes. This is also true for most people who, like Walter, believe they would desire assisted suicide.

In a society where laws protect individual rights, we sometimes lose sight of the impact of our actions upon others, particularly those who love us. When faced with the complexity of the issue and given the opportunity to live the last weeks and months of life in comfort with loved ones near by, the decision to continue living is the characteristic choice.

Perhaps we are not asking the right questions in approaching the important discussions about end-of-life decision-making. Addressing fears and ensuring adequate pain- and symptom-management seem paramount. Individual quality-of-life concerns deserve concerted attention and efforts to address them. The question that logically and morally emerges, then, is when will comprehensive, humane hospice care and services be available to all people who are dying?

> *In the last analysis, it is our conception of death which decides our answers to all the questions that life puts to us. That is why it requires its proper place and time if need be, with right of precedence. Hence, too, the necessity of preparing for it.*
>
> —DAG HAMMARSKJOLD
> *MARKINGS* [13]

Chapter Six

THE HEART HAS REASONS
What It Means to Be a
Hospice Volunteer

**Columbia Hospice Volunteer and
Team Training Program**

SESSION FOUR: "The Role of the Volunteer in Hospice
and Working with Diversity in Hospice Families"
THURSDAY, APRIL 25TH, 7–9 P.M.
PANEL OF SPEAKERS: Gertrude Marcinek, Louise Guiterez, Marion Waters, and Martin Steinberg

Barbara Murphy (Columbia Hospice Coordinator of Volunteers): Good evening and welcome to this week's session of our hospice's volunteer and team training. Tonight we will explore the role of the hospice volunteer and look at working with racial, cultural, and religious differences. To begin the evening we have invited a panel of Columbia Hospice volunteers to speak with you about what it means to be a hospice volunteer. I would like to introduce the panelists to you: Gertrude Marcinek, who will talk about what brings people to volunteer for hospice; Louise Guiterez, who will tell you about her experience of working on hospice's inpatient unit; Marion Waters, who will address working with families of different racial, cultural, or religious backgrounds; and Martin Steinberg, who will discuss his experience as a bereavement volunteer. All of these volunteers will speak from the vantage point of their actual experiences in working with hospice families. Because of the importance of maintaining the families' confidentiality, all the family names have been changed. Following the panel's presentation, you will have the opportunity to ask questions. We will then take a short break and you will be involved in a small-group activity that explores the reasons you have for volunteering with hospice. Thank you very much, Gertrude, Louise, Marion, and Martin, for generously agreeing to present tonight.

Gertrude Marcinek: My name is Gertrude Marcinek and I've been a volunteer with Columbia Hospice for the past year and a half. I've been asked today to tell you the story of how I became involved with hospice. My mother died three years ago this May. Congestive heart failure held her in its grip for at least ten years and during that time she lost more and more of her strength. In spite of constant medical attention, that last year she just couldn't seem to stabilize. The medications she took always needed adjusting or changing, and her weariness grew and clouded her days.

I marveled that her spunk and wit still sparked as she put up with her increasing limitations and physical problems. During the last six years of her life she had two major heart attacks and was resuscitated once after her heart stopped. She had no regrets about the resuscitation. In fact, during it she'd had a religious vision. Things changed for Mom after that. She said she was less afraid and that she would be ready to go when her time came. When Dr. Gibson told my mother that her condition was becoming less and less responsive to the medications, my mother was quick to let her know that she was not interested in trying anything new. She told her, "I'm

86 and I've lived a rich life. It's time to just let nature take its course without too much fuss."

After a conversation about the available treatment options, my mother asked Dr. Gibson what would happen if they did not pursue any additional treatments. Dr. Gibson began by telling my mother that her heart was not keeping up with the day-to-day demands, and wasn't pumping efficiently enough to keep her body working. Medications would continue to help somewhat with the fluid retention and the shortness of breath, but it was becoming more and more difficult to keep up with the problems. Then Dr. Gibson asked my mother what kind of care she wanted.

Mom was definite when she said that she didn't want many more treatments or procedures, and that she definitely did not want to be resuscitated again. Dr. Gibson said that it was time to talk about specifics. She suggested we meet with the office nurse about the paperwork involved for a living will and advance directives. It was helpful for me to be there with my mother when we were talking with the doctor about her wishes. Dr. Gibson reassured my mother that she would follow through on her choices regarding treatment. Then she called in the nurse and we spoke with her and set up a follow-up appointment for two weeks later.

Talking about the end of a life is never easy, especially when it's about someone you love. My mother and I spent long hours in conversation. We called my cousin who is an attorney in Chicago and he sent along forms for a durable power of attorney that we had notarized at the bank. Together we filled out the living will, the do-not-resuscitate, and the advance directives forms and signed them. I was surprised about how certain Mom was about no extraordinary measures. In all the situations listed, she only wanted to be kept comfortable. By the next visit with Dr. Gibson, my mother had completed all her paperwork. Those conversations helped me understand what was important to my mother. During those talks we said important things to each other. They made the months ahead easier.

By the way, I know that all of you received copies of these forms in your information packet. I would strongly encourage you to look at them and complete them with your family member's and give copies of them to your family physician.

Anyway, I'll continue with my story. Everyone who knew my mother would describe her as strong and independent. Until two months before she died she lived in her own home, a five-minute drive from our house. I visited her every day, taking her groceries and an occasional meal.

Most of Mom's friends were already gone, but some of the younger people in the neighborhood would call and visit. And I know her five grandchildren kept in close touch with her. My mother was a well-loved woman.

Between the time she spoke to Dr. Gibson about her wishes and the time of her death, five months passed. Her weakness weighed her down those last months. And, at the end, her breath was so short that she had to stop five or six times on her way to the bathroom. It wasn't easy to convince her to come live with us, but she knew she just couldn't manage things alone any longer. My husband, Joe, helped move her in and made her feel welcome.

Mom admitted that she had been lonely at her home sometimes. Now she worried that she was too much trouble for us. That's when Dr. Gibson referred us to hospice. Before then I had never heard of hospice, though Mom said hospice had cared for her neighbor, Mrs. Smolarek, the previous year. Mom was pleased with her hospice nurse, Catherine. A nursing assistant, Jean, came three times a week to help Mom and they teased and joked a lot together.

One person we all liked from hospice was the volunteer, Josephine. Jo came every Tuesday and Thursday morning to visit my mother. She and Mom had both grown up in the same town in northern Michigan and they both had been widowed more than a dozen years ago. Jo was eighteen years younger than my mother, but they had a lot in common. They would sit and talk for hours, telling each other stories. When Mom was too weak or short of breath, Jo would read to her, or they would watch TV together. I will always remember the look of anticipation on Mom's face when Jo walked in the door. Jo is one of those people you just feel comfortable around.

Dr. Gibson was good about seeing Mom every month, adjusting her medications and offering her some special attention. It was the Monday after Mother's Day when Mom started to have chest pain, and I took her to Dr. Gibson's that morning. She'd had a bad cold for the past week. After a thorough examination, Dr. Gibson told us that Mom had pneumonia in both lungs. Dr. Gibson talked with my mother about starting on antibiotics, but Mom was immovable. Finally, Dr. Gibson accepted my mother's decision. She acknowledged that my mother had been feeling poorly for quite a while. Promising my mother that she would do all she could to keep her comfortable, Dr. Gibson ordered oxygen and some new medications through hospice. Before we left, Dr. Gibson offered that if my mother changed her mind about the antibiotics, or if she needed anything· else, we should call. She said that she would stay in close contact with the hospice nurse and reassured us that hospice would be able to offer us the kind of support we would need. Dr. Gibson even offered to make a house call. My mother thanked her for all her help, and all the extra time and attention, and for respecting her wishes.

When the hospice nurse, Catherine, arrived that afternoon, she had already arranged for the oxygen Dr. Gibson had ordered to be delivered. She sat and talked specifics with Mom and me for a while, telling us that Mom probably wouldn't last more than a week. The oxygen helped Mom's breathing, and she enjoyed sitting in the recliner in the living room those first two days. Barbara, the hospice nursing assistant, came in every morning that week, and Jo sat with Mom for an hour each afternoon so I could rest. Our parish priest came on Thursday evening to give Mom the last rites. I remember how she smiled after he finished.

Mom died Saturday evening. Though she was unresponsive for the last forty-eight hours, I know that she was at peace with her life. At about midnight she just slowly stopped breathing. I was relieved not to have her in the hospital with all the machines. When she went, I was sitting right by her bed, with my hand resting gently on her arm.

When I think back on it, it still seems strange. I'm 57 years old and my mother was always there for me. Now she's gone. It was so hard to see her diminished and unable to do the things she enjoyed those last few years. When we talked after her last visit to Dr. Gibson, Mom told me that 86 years was a lot of time and that she wasn't afraid to die. She told me it would have been different if she'd felt better. The main thing that made her dying tolerable for her was the religious experience that she had had when she was resuscitated. She believed that she was going to see God. When she died, there was a sense of peacefulness about it. I miss her and all that we shared. It's strange to know that both my parents are gone now. I'm not sure I like being the older generation.

A few months after Mom's death, I received a second call from the hospice bereavement volunteer who had visited me a few weeks after Mom died. I told her that I was doing pretty well, except for the fact that I felt at loose ends sometimes. When I no longer had Mom to care for, I began delivering meals-on-wheels twice a week. I was glad the volunteer called, because I had been thinking about volunteering for hospice. She told me that hospice would be happy to have my help when a year had passed since Mom's death.

That year went by quickly. I realize that keeping busy and helping others are ways that I cope. After the anniversary of my mother's death, I called Barbara, the coordinator of volunteers here at Columbia Hospice and scheduled an interview. I was accepted as a hospice volunteer and attended the volunteer training program the next fall. As you know, it was a moving and powerful learning experience. That fall I started working with hospice as a home-care volunteer.

I'm sure that many of you have similar family stories and experiences that brought you to hospice. I wanted to be part of a group of people who were so caring and helpful to families at a time when they truly needed it. I don't know when I've ever met finer people than the hospice staff and the families we serve. The people who are dying and their families are in such tender and fragile times. I wanted to give to others some of the wonderful support I received around Mom's death. When I think about my volunteer work with hospice during the past year and a half, I realize what an important part of my life it has become. I feel very lucky to be involved with hospice and welcome all of you to this fine organization.

Louise Guiterez: Good evening. I'm Louise Guiterez and I have been a volunteer on the Colombia Hospice inpatient unit for the past two years. I have been asked to speak about a special experience I have had working as a volunteer on the unit. You will all take a tour of the unit before the end of the training. There are eight beds on the unit, and most of the patients there are quite ill. Some of them are transferred from the hospital and some are admitted from home for special care of pain or symptoms. Most patients stay one to three days on the unit. Almost a third of the patients who are admitted to the unit die there. So, inpatient unit volunteers learn to handle brief contacts with patients and families in a time of great need.

I am 66 years old and retired and I live in the neighborhood near the hospital. Two days a week I volunteer on the inpatient unit. I have a big family here in the city, so the rest of my time I spend with them and volunteering at Sacred Heart Church. Hospice is important to me and I find my work here like a prayer: I send it out and hope that it will do some good. Columbia Hospice helped us care for my cousin

Juanita when she died of leukemia three years ago. I think that's why I want to tell you about the Ferris family.

Joel Ferris and his family were very loving people. Joel was transferred to the hospice inpatient unit after his bone marrow transplant failed. He was only 20 years old, and his parents and sister stayed with him the entire two days he was on the unit. When I talked with Joel he wanted more than anything to go home. Joel was so weak and yet we all believed he would make it home. His parents were working with the home-care team to make it happen. Joel slipped into a coma the next night and died the following afternoon. His parents and his sister, Amy were with Joel when he died, and I could tell that it was unbelievably terrible for them to let him go. For a year they had followed every treatment that the doctors recommended. They did everything and nothing worked. Joel died only eleven months after he had been diagnosed with leukemia.

My memory tends to hold pictures, sort of like my own personal snapshots of moments or images that are special to me. The pictures that stay with me most of the Ferris family are about the way that they were with each other. The first image that I remember is how they looked when they came on the unit that first morning. I knew that everyone was afraid, and that they weren't sure hospice was the right place. After Joel was settled in the room, the family started bringing in his things. In a short while, the room was full of photos, posters, cards, stuffed animals, a tennis racket and balls, a favorite quilt, a radio and tape player, and books.

The family began telling me stories about Joel, his treatments, and about the years before the leukemia. Joel had a friendly sense of humor and he entertained us with his stories and jokes, too. That's the image I hold, of the family smiling and telling anecdotes about the young man they loved and about each other.

Then I remember the morning that Joel died. The mental picture of his sister, Amy, cuddled on top of his bed next to him is one I will never forget. They had the kind of closeness that is unique for a brother and sister, and were less than two years apart in age. Amy had the tape player on and she was singing some of their favorite songs to Joel. I'm not up on popular music, but it was some kind of folk rock, with tender, sad words. It fit perfectly.

After Joel died that afternoon, I remained with the family. Mrs. Ferris's sister arrived and they all stayed with Joel's body. It was almost a sacred ritual the way they were saying good-bye to this young man they loved so dearly. I found myself crying, too. My people cry easily, especially when someone dies—even the men. I could feel love in the room both days that I was with the family. Not all families show that much love.

I didn't know what the word "bereft" meant until I was with the Ferris family. I can't imagine what it would be like to lose a child, or to lose your only brother. The Ferrises will still have a lot of love for each other, but Joel's death must have left an unbelievable hole in their lives.

A few days afterward I wrote the Ferris family a note. The family also sent a thank-you letter to the hospice inpatient unit. They said how much they appreciated my staying with them when Joel was dying. Amy said I was just like her grandma would have been if she had been there. That meant a lot to me. I never saw them again, but I have my pictures that will stay with me. Working with hospice shows us some very painful things, but it also shows us the best in people. God bless you all in your volunteer work with hospice.

Marion Waters: Hello. My name is Marion Waters. I'm pleased to be here this evening, and a little nervous, too. I've been a volunteer with Columbia Hospice for just over a year.

I became interested in hospice after I heard Barbara speak at our church about hospice's need for volunteers. Tonight, she has asked me to tell you about my experience as an African-American volunteer, and to speak to the issue of working with people of different races, backgrounds, cultures, or religions. I notice she put together a diverse panel here that represents many of the people we care for at Columbia Hospice. I'm not an expert on cultural considerations, but I have worked through to an understanding of some basic suggestions that I would like to offer to you tonight.

Because Barbara asked us to use actual stories when we spoke, I decided that I would tell you about the five weeks that I visited Frances Johnson. The Johnsons were the first family that I worked with as a hospice volunteer. Frances was a 49-year-old widow who worked at the local auto plant. Six months before Dr. Wong at City General referred Frances to hospice, she was diagnosed with breast cancer. In fact, for some time Frances had noticed a sore on her breast that was growing and had waited to see a doctor. She prayed that it would go away. By the time of her surgery, the cancer had spread to her lymph nodes. For the next six weeks she went for radiation treatments and continued to work. The three-month follow-up X ray showed that the cancer had begun to spread to her lungs and she was referred to hospice.

The first time I visited Frances Johnson, she was still living in her own apartment. Frances was a quiet but friendly woman who loved singing in the church choir. Since she had been ill, she'd missed most of the choir practices and half of the Sunday services. Frances's sister, Mary, and her family lived two blocks away. Frances was very close to her sister's family and spent a lot of time with her two nieces and her nephew.

I learned that Frances's husband, Bobby, had been killed in Vietnam, and that she had never remarried. Frances had a number of friends and she prided herself in having been a member of the church choir for fifteen years. She openly talked about how the Lord had helped her through the dark times

. after Bobby died and that she knew he would help her now.

One of the strange parts of being a hospice volunteer is not knowing how the person who is ill or the family will react to you, what they will find helpful. With Frances, as it has been with most of the hospice families I've worked with, mostly I've been a listener, offering companionship and being there for people in small ways.

One important thing that I did with Frances was help her arrange the times friends and choir members would come by so she wouldn't be alone so much during the day. Mary and the children spent a lot of time with Frances in the evenings. When Frances got so weak she couldn't manage on her own, she moved in with Mary and her family. Frances didn't want to leave her place, but she knew it would make things easier on Mary to have Frances there.

I visited Frances over at Mary's, especially during the day. Frances had a lot of people who cared about her, and they came by and brought meals regularly. It was hard for Frances because she didn't have much energy or breath to talk a lot. She always got her strength up when Pastor Freeman came to visit, usually twice a week. They prayed together, and he usually sang with Frances, too.

One day Frances said that she had asked the nurse how much longer this would go on. The nurse told Frances that she couldn't say for sure, but that when Frances's time came, she would know it, and would feel more ready then. Frances prayed that was true. She still wanted to be well more than anything. Whenever she had strength, she read the Bible, searching for words of comfort. Sometimes I read the Bible to Frances during my visit.

Before she had left her apartment, Frances asked me to put some of her things in a box and bring them to Mary's. She asked me to bring her two photo albums, Bobby's Purple Heart and Silver Star from Vietnam, his gold watch, and a silver pin that had been her mother's. She had me put her toolbox in another box and take it, too. During the next few days she began giving her family the things in those boxes. She gave

Bobby's medals to Tom, her 13-year-old nephew, and told him his uncle would have been as proud as she was of the man he was becoming. That same evening she gave her 16-year-old niece Sandra the silver pin that was her grandmother's, telling her that she had her grandmother's same strong spirit. Frances gave her Bible to Angela, her 11-year-old niece. She asked Angela to read to her from it once in a while. Angela said "I don't want you to go." Frances responded with, "I don't want to go either, Angela. We all need to answer when the Lord calls us. Even if we don't like it."

Frances gave her brother-in-law, Lamar, the toolbox that had been Bobby's. Then she gave Mary her two albums. One had pictures from their childhood and of the time with Bobby. It also had the letters he sent Frances from Vietnam in it. The second album was of the recent years and had all the pictures and cards the children had made for her. She told Mary that she wanted her to have all her special things so that Mary would remember all the good times and the love they'd shared.

The following Monday when Ella, the hospice nursing assistant, came to bathe Frances, she noticed how much she was failing. Ella often sang to Frances when she was caring for her, and this morning Frances chose "Eagle's Wings."

Mary told me that the next morning Frances had motioned to her to lean close. Frances whispered that she had seen Bobby the night before smiling and looking handsome. He told Frances he was waiting for her. Mary said she told Frances that Bobby certainly had loved her a great deal, and that he probably was waiting for her. Mary knew that Frances's time was short and she stayed home from work the next few days. Frances passed on Thursday.

I wasn't surprised when I went to the funeral to see how large it was. The choir sang some of Frances's favorite hymns. When we sang "Amazing Grace," I felt tears for the loss of this sweet soul, Frances, and for all the people I had lost, too.

The next week I went to see Mary and her family one last time, to say good-bye. Mary told me that the nurse had come by to pick up the equipment and visited for a while. I told Mary that they were the first family I had worked with in hospice, and how much it had meant to me to meet them. Mary thanked me and said she and Frances had always felt at home with me. I suppose that's the best thing anyone can say to a hospice volunteer.

Now, about the differences we see in each other. Differences can create misunderstandings and sometimes judgments. The one thing I would say to you is to be very careful in your hospice volunteering not to judge people. If you don't know or don't understand something that a family says or does, ask them about their patterns. We usually like to tell people about the things that are important to us.

I know that you have some materials in you packet about the ways different races, cultures, and religions deal with death. The important thing is to treat people like individuals, and with respect for their own ways and beliefs.

In the African-American tradition, as well as for many other minority cultures, including Mexican-American and Jewish people, extended family and kinship networks are very important. Minority people have learned to stand together and look after their own. There is sometimes mistrust of authority or systems where people believe they have no power. For example, that may be one of the reasons why Frances waited too long before seeking care.

When in doubt, ask the family what is important to them. Frances told me how important her faith was to her. It gave her strength to face her illness and dying. And the story Mary told me about Frances saying she saw Bobby is similar to ones I have heard since then from other patients. I don't question them, I just listen. We don't need to understand or agree with everything that goes on with the hospice families that we work with. It just seems important to honor them and their experiences.

All families have strengths, so be sure to recognize and acknowledge the family's strengths. Sometimes it may be important for you as a volunteer to be an advocate for the family with the hospice professionals, especially if there is a misunderstanding or if some medical or nursing care is not clear to them.

Finally, look at the family's beliefs and the importance of religion or a religious community. The church was at the heart of Frances's support. Volunteers need to work with the existing support of the family.

The way I see my volunteering is that death humbles us all, and makes us aware of all that we don't know and can't do. That same principle is true for your work with minority families. Be respectful and humble and let them tell you what is important. Honor their ways of doing things. Good luck to you all.

Martin Steinberg: Hello. I'm Martin Steinberg. I've been a volunteer with Columbia Hospice for a year and a half, and before that I worked with hospice for a year as a student intern during my masters in social work program at the university. When I was an intern, I worked in all areas of hospice: home care, the hospital inpatient unit, the nursing home wing at Portland Place, and in the bereavement program. Now I'm employed by social services in the city, and for the past year and a half I have been a bereavement volunteer. Two years ago, I was asked to visit Mr. Hyman Cohen and do a bereavement assessment after Rebecca, his wife of forty-nine years, died of uterine cancer.

Hyman was a well-respected retired engineer who held several patents for his work. Rebecca was a teacher, and for the last twenty years of her life volunteered at the local high school. They were both involved in civic affairs and served on a number of community boards before Rebecca became seriously ill.

Hospice was involved for only two weeks before Mrs.

Cohen's death. The nurse and nursing assistant were concerned about Mr. Cohen because of his history and because he was now alone. I want to tell you about my first meeting with Hyman Cohen, and the stories I heard from him later.

The Cohens lost many members of their family during the Holocaust. Hyman was the youngest of three children, and his two sisters and parents died in a concentration camp in Poland. Hyman managed to escape and came to the U.S., where he served in the army for the remainder of the war.

After the war ended he met Rebecca, and they married the next year. Mr. Cohen told me that their love meant all the more to them since they had lost so much of their family. Their first child, Judith, died when she was three months old of what we know now as sudden infant death syndrome (SIDS). Two years later they had a son, David, who has lived in Haifa, Israel, since he was 27. David is now in his early forties and is married with a son who is 8 and a 6-year-old daughter. While David has a tender relationship with his father, the great distance means that there is little practical help he can offer him. Rebecca and Hyman used to travel to Israel once a year to see David and his family.

Hyman and Rebecca had many friends, and were involved in the Jewish community. While they were never highly religious, being Jewish was an essential part of their identity and their world. Each year they attended high holiday services but did not participate regularly in synagogue activities.

I was concerned about Mr. Cohen, now 84, and his many losses and his aloneness. Isolation is considered a major risk factor for grieving persons. Mr. Cohen's life had held a great deal of sorrow. He did have numerous friends, though, and I soon learned that his approach to life was a spirited one. I kept in contact with Mr. Cohen, by phone mostly, for the following year. He was not interested in attending any of the bereavement support groups, preferring instead the company and comfort of his friends.

I saw Mr. Cohen again six months ago when he was

admitted to our hospice inpatient unit. I was visiting the unit to meet with the staff for the biweekly meeting to discuss the recent deaths and bereavement referrals. When I learned that Mr. Cohen had been admitted, I stopped by to see him. He looked very pale and thinner than the last time we met. He was only 5'6" tall, and lying in bed made him seem even smaller. In advanced stages of lymphoma, he was experiencing major weakness and some pain. Mr. Cohen would be transferred to our hospice wing at Portland Manor nursing home after his symptoms were stabilized.

It struck me as sad that this man who had been so faithful in his wife's care was now alone. Though he was weak, Mr. Cohen was cheerful and his courtesy reminded me of the formality of European social graces. Something in his manner was both dignified and friendly. It didn't take long for me to realize again what a striking and charming gentleman this was.

Shortly after his admission, Mr. Cohen was given a blood transfusion to build up his strength. He was willing to have the transfusion in the hopes of having enough energy to enjoy his son's visit in ten days. The second reason why he had agreed to the transfusion was because he was scheduled for his Shoah interview the day after tomorrow. The Shoah interviews are a special project started by a famous American filmmaker to record on tape and film the stories of Holocaust survivors. Mr. Cohen told his doctor that this would be his last transfusion.

After Mr. Cohen told me about his Shoah interview, he asked if I would be with him when the interview took place. He decided to go ahead with the scheduled interview, and the hospice social worker phoned and arranged for it to be held in Mr. Cohen's room on the hospice unit late the following afternoon. I felt pleased that Mr. Cohen had asked me and I agreed to be there with him during the interview.

Hearing Hyman Cohen's story moved me deeply. Because I am Jewish, I have been interested in stories of the Holocaust. But I had never heard a personal account like Mr. Cohen's troubling and remarkable story of survival. I felt only the deepest admiration for this man who had endured so much and was still so alive and engaged with life. Afterward he asked the interviewers if hospice could have a copy of the tape, too.

The following day Mr. Cohen went to the hospice unit at Portland Place. I saw him there once more, just after his son returned to Israel. He died three weeks after he went to the nursing home hospice wing. I still think of him. When I pass the room he was in in the inpatient unit, where the interview took place, I hear parts of his story again in my mind. His life was marked by significant sorrows and yet he never became bitter. Sometimes he said he withdrew into himself, but when I think of Hyman Cohen I see him smiling and talking. People who have known grief seem to live life differently. Hyman stayed a caring, involved person until his life ended.

Hospice work reminds me of what life is about, of the wonders of the human heart and the human spirit. I have learned a great deal from the people I work with. I know that, unlike Mr. Cohen, some of them have not always been the nicest people, or the most attentive family members. But dying can bring the best in people to the surface. It gives families opportunities to be together in new and different ways. The process of dying and the act of caregiving can create a new reality, easing the burden of past difficulties. I especially like working with grieving family members. Grief involves so much sorrow and searching. The bereaved people I work with are so grateful for hospice's continuing contact, and for the information and support we offer. It's a very important part of hospice volunteering. I hope that all of you find your hospice work as inspiring as I have.

No one is as capable of gratitude as one who has emerged from the kingdom of night. We know that every moment is a moment of grace, every hour an offering; not to share them would mean to betray them. Our lives no longer belong to us alone; they belong to all those who need us desperately.

—ELIE WIESEL

Hospice Volunteers

Hospice volunteers are often considered the heart of a hospice program and its services. They are among a hospice's most valued and appreciated resources. Many hospice volunteers come to work in a hospice following a personal experience with the death of a loved one. They have a sincere desire to help others who are facing difficult times. Other people volunteer for hospice to maintain a healthy perspective on their own lives and losses, drawing upon the compassion and understanding their personal experiences have generated.

Typically, prospective volunteers contact a hospice program and express interest in becoming involved. The coordinator of volunteers gives potential volunteers written information about hospice and its various programs, and asks them to complete an application. After the completed application form is received, the hospice coordinator of volunteers sets up an interview to meet with the interested individual to discuss hospice involvement.

Just as there are selection criteria for hospice professionals, there are basic qualities that are desirable in hospice volunteers. Volunteer coordinators look for individuals who have sources of internal strength and external support. Feelings of acceptance, mutual respect, and positive regard or liking that are characteristics of helping relationships also are important in the hospice volunteer. Finally, idealism, altruism, and the capacity for empathy build the bridge of the helping relationship between the hospice volunteer and the family.[1]

Sustaining Relationships

Perhaps the overriding selection criteria for hospice volunteers involve the qualities valued most by people who are dying and grieving. Several characteristics and abilities define *sustaining relationships:*[2]

Presence   Because words are so inadequate or incomplete, there are no words that can take a person's pain or distress away. We say so much of what we mean through our nonverbal communication (65–90 percent). Perhaps the greatest gift that we give another person is to be with them, to stand with them in difficult times.

Ability to Listen / Empathy   Few of us have enough people who will listen to us in an open, noncritical way. In difficult times, there is a great need to talk about one's experience, to review the details, to tell one's story. Most people listen with the goal of giving answers or advice. The pure yet difficult gift of genuinely listening allows the person speaking to see and understand his experience in an expanded way. People feel understood and comforted when we try to empathize and enter into their world. When we try to understand what it might be like to be in the other person's place, it can diminish his or her feelings of distress or isolation.

Life Experience / Maturity   We are the product of our own experiences and of our reactions to them. Our experiences, both positive and difficult, teach us about the world and other people. Maturity is the ability to integrate and use those experiences in a way that not only increases our understanding, but also enhances our personal power and our compassion.

Comfort   When we are in the midst of a difficult time, it is helpful to be around people who are comfortable with emotions and with their role as a helping person. Most of all, we appreciate people who are comfortable with themselves, who try to live with the reality of human and life limitations, and who are able to offer comfort to others.

Interpersonal Skills   There is a way of being with others that gives them the impression that they matter, and that you have nothing else to do at that moment. The better ways of responding to people in difficult times involve using our best communication skills to honor the person's responses and abilities. Trust is an essential ingredient in relationships because it conveys belief in the person, and in his or her eventual ability to cope.

Caring / Concern   Like love, caring is a small word that attempts to convey a large experience. Caring involves warmth and acceptance of another person that is expressed in the relationship. There is a sense of kindness, gentleness, and concern for the well-being of another that comforts and sustains us in difficult and good times. We offer and receive caring in personal relationships and in our larger human community, out of our understanding that what happens to another person matters.

Compassion   The ability to sit with and fully acknowledge the experience of a person in a painful time is a remarkable capacity that is born out of a personal understanding of our own struggles and of the human condition. Compassion is the most profound level of human caring.

Patience   We all struggle to cope with difficult times in our own ways, and in our own time. And for everyone, difficult times seem too slow, or too long. Coping with major changes involves an ongoing series of adaptations, and is a process that takes significant energy and time. People know when we feel that they are not moving quickly enough. Relationships where there is a commitment to journey with a person through difficult times are both necessary and invaluable.

Sensitivity   In responding to others in times of their need, we often try to offer traditional wisdoms, or clichés that we have heard before. It is important not to say things that only comfort us, and might create distress for the other person. Sensitivity also means being aware of cues that will allow us to anticipate the needs of the person.

Courage   The strength to face our own difficulties and those of people we care about is not an inborn trait. We are not born brave; it is a quality we develop when we creatively enter into the full range of human experience. We choose to face our difficulties and to be present with others in theirs because we are asked to, because it is needed or required of us in the situation. Courage is an act of generosity of the spirit for ourselves and for those that we care about.

Volunteer Training Programs

All hospice volunteers attend a volunteer training and/or a team training program that the hospice offers. These training programs are generally offered two to four times each year and consist of at least twenty-two hours of information. Many hospices offer programs that comprise as many as forty hours of training. Topics covered in the hospice volunteer training include:

- Introduction to hospice care and principles
- The role of the volunteer in hospice
- Concepts of death and dying
- Communication skills
- Care and comfort measures
- Diseases and medical conditions
- Psychosocial and spiritual concerns related to dying
- Family-centered care
- Interdisciplinary teamwork
- Stress management
- Grief and support during bereavement
- Safety and infection control
- Confidentiality and patients' rights[3]

Following the volunteer training program, volunteers become involved visiting hospice families in their homes and in hospice facilities such as inpatient units, nursing homes, or a hospice residential facility. Hospice volunteers contribute to the plan of care and communicate with other members of the interdisciplinary team. There are also hospice volunteers who offer bereavement care and services, and others who assist in office work and fund-raising efforts.

Rewards of Hospice Volunteers

John Brantner, a psychologist involved in the early development of hospice care, believed that the major lessons we learn from people who are dying concern the importance of openness and sharing ourselves more freely in our relationships. He believed that our personal growth comes from the outside and depends on relationships.[4] Hospice care offers a unique model of caring relationships.

Volunteers and professionals involved with hospice care typically report high levels of satisfaction with their work. Most volunteers feel they get back more than they give to others. They seem to value the understandings that working with people who are dying and grieving bring into their own lives. Above all, they treasure the privilege of sharing in hospice families' most tender times.

> *The miracle is this—the more we share, the more we have.*
>
> —LEONARD NIMOY

Minority Cultures: Illness and Dying

Illness and death take place in a personal context that is shaped by our culture, our religious beliefs, and our community. These influences create our reality, defining the ways that we view or appraise death and grief. They also form the rules that we learned about acceptable emotional responses to these critical life experiences. Finally, cultural and religious affiliations influence the crucial element of social support.

Hospices across the country began their programs by offering services to families who were like the early volunteers: white, middle class, primarily Christian people. While there were no efforts to exclude or deny services to minorities, there was little consciousness about the needs of dying persons and their families in minority communities.

Hospice's lack of services to minority cultures is reflective of the gaps that exist throughout the health care system and other systems in our society. In fact, the experience of being part of a minority group involves dealing with deficits. Bridging these deficits of opportunity, access, acceptance, and understanding are particularly important when minority culture families are facing the complicated experience of life-threatening illness and death.

Dr. Howard Wilson of Harvard University addressed the Institute on Education in Human Relations in Cleveland, Ohio, and offered fours ways of improving intergroup relations:

1. More information, facts, and more objective experience in intercultural relations
2. Some means for sympathetic communication with other people
3. Some means for better understanding of other people
4. Exploration of whole new areas of experience through the much-needed medium of shared conversation[5]

These recommendations, made fifty years ago, have direct application to the extension of hospice services to minority cultures. They mirror our best current efforts at diversity training and understanding. The National Hospice Organization's *Standards of a Hospice Program of Care* and its *Task Force on Access to Hospice Care by Minorities* both recognize the importance of specific efforts aimed at providing the highest quality services to diverse populations.

Barriers to Access of Hospice Services

In recent years, at both the national and the community level, there has been a recognition that minority groups have had limited access to hospice services. Significant barriers to providing services to minority cultures have been identified at all levels: the professional health care referral sources, hospice providers, the hospice staff members, and minority families themselves.

People of color are highly aware of "second class" treatment, and may be skeptical about the quality of hospice services, perceiving that the care may be less desirable than hospital care. Others may fear that selecting hospice services excludes them from the acute-care system. Some minority or ethnic groups may also see hospice services as removed from their needs and concerns, geographically or practically. Minority families have difficulty trusting health care providers, or the system in general. Other barriers include lack of knowledge, fear, alienation, hopelessness, and lack of ability to identify with providers.[6]

Trust was a concern in Frances Johnson's reluctance to seek medical treatment when her tumor first appeared. Lacking a consistent relationship with a physician, Frances was fearful of seeking medical help. Even the long wait typical of the university or city outpatient clinics can be a deterrent. Mistrust and cultural factors are also logical influences in decisions not to pursue experimental treatments.

Other more concrete fears of minority populations include suspicion surrounding medical forms, having strangers in the home, and fear of the discovery of an illegal immigrant family member in the home. Or, family members may see involvement with hospice care as "giving up" on the ill family member.[7]

Hospices and Access

Physicians and other health care professionals are a major source of information about hospice care, as well as referrals. Many of the health care professionals who serve minority community members lack knowledge of hospice care or of the ways to access hospice services. Hospices and health care professionals share responsibility to ensure that information about hospice services is available to all those people who could benefit from them.

The providers of hospice services need to know about cultural diversity, and need to have staff members and volunteers representing minority populations. Most importantly, the core hospice caregiving qualities of a nonjudgmental approach, openness, sensitivity, and the willingness to learn from the families themselves will provide the means for the best possible care and services.[8]

Families from minority cultural backgrounds are similar in some ways to all families, and different in other unique ways. About one hundred identifiable ethnic groups have been recognized in the United States.[9] There can be a tendency for health care providers to view these groups as homogeneous, treating them in similar ways. Each ethnic group and the subcultures within it have differences and reflect a particular history and social background. Respectful, knowledgeable attention to the ways that hospice services can be shaped to meet the needs of minority communities is an important goal. Achieving this goal will take continued commitment, planning, outreach, and education. The important words of Dame Cicely Saunders, the designer of the modern hospice movement, apply directly to concerns about serving minority populations. The principle of valuing and respecting the life of all dying persons is inherent in her words: "You matter because you are you. You matter to the last moment of your life, and we will do all we can, not only to help you die in peace, but also to live until you die."[10]

Chapter Seven

IF WISHES WERE HORSES
A Girl's Special Relationship with
Her Sick Mother

KATHY LOVED THE sloping fields and grasses outside of town. She walked there to look at the horses every chance that she could. Now that her mother was getting sicker, she didn't get out there as much. Everything was changing for Kathy and her mother, and it wasn't getting better.

When the days were hard, Kathy wished that she knew where her dad was. It was nine years since he left, and she had only the thinnest memories, mostly shaped by the few photos her mother had given her. Why did he leave them? Why was her mother so sick? Sometimes Kathy felt so afraid that she just shut off thinking about things. Maybe her mother would get better soon.

Wanda worried about Kathy. For the twelve years of her life, she had been a quiet girl, helpful and never one to complain much. That was probably because it was just the two of them. After Joe left, Wanda found work cleaning houses and then got on at the furniture plant in town. It was just about the only place to work in Greenville. Their life had finally evened out and felt steady. Like most single parents, Wanda relied heavily on Kathy to assume some of the household responsibilities. There just aren't many choices when you're raising a child alone.

In the fall last year, Wanda felt so poorly that she decided to go to the doctor. The look on the doctor's face when he set up the appointment for her to go to the specialist told her that things were bad. Then the specialist did the biopsy and found the cancer. He said it was melanoma, one of the worst kinds of cancer, and it had already spread. It had started with the growth on her back. For a while, Wanda hadn't seen it or known it was there. Then, she thought that it was probably something that would go away. When it didn't, she began to worry. If she hadn't felt so bad, she would never have gone to the doctor. Why should she go just to get a mole taken off? After all, no one could see it anyway.

Wanda began to worry about Kathy. Who would take care of her if something happened? It never occurred to Wanda that she would be in this spot. She saw herself as a young, strong woman. She always figured that if she got through that bad time after Joe had left, her life would be okay.

When the doctors gave Wanda such small odds of the treatments working, she decided not to have any. "I've never been very good at gambling, or at beating the odds. And less than 15 percent in the best of situations is not much of a chance." Why should she put herself through all that, and have all the expense besides? Wanda did have surgery to remove the growth on her back. The doctors hoped that it might slow down the spread. They went pretty deep, but eventually the spot had healed.

Wanda's friend at work, Violet, had taken her husband to see a healer when he had bladder cancer. So far he was still doing well, and that was over two years ago. Twila Starr was not a doctor, but she had studied Native American and Chinese healing practices. Her mother had been a well-known healer in the area. The biggest problem with seeing Twila Starr was that she lived fifty miles away, and most of it over country roads. The trip took the better part of two hours each way. Wanda went on Saturdays for two months, with Kathy along.

Wanda and Kathy talked about the feeling of peace in

Twila's place. Twila laid her hands on Wanda's back and ribs every time that they went. When Twila put her hands on Wanda's head and held them there for what seemed like ten minutes, Wanda saw a purple round shape with a gold center, edged with shimmering green. It moved and changed in and out like a kaleidoscope. Wanda never told Twila, but it was so calming and lifted her spirits. It was what she looked forward to most on their visits. That, and just being in her place, which seemed like a haven.

Twila Starr gave Wanda herbs to take four times a day. The process of boiling and preparing the herbs was something Kathy did every morning, before she left for school. Kathy felt sick to her stomach when she cooked the herbs. They smelled so awful. She didn't complain, and instead just tried to air out the house after her mother left for work, and opened the windows again after school. The smell wouldn't matter so much if her mother got better. Kathy liked Twila Starr and trusted her.

Wanda was still working at the plant, but she was calling in sick about once a week, and came home early a few times. She told her supervisor, and he was trying to help her out and cover for her. This week they talked about her going on leave, or filing for the disability benefit. It would take two months before it went into effect, so it might be wise to consider stopping work now. The people at work were so friendly and helpful that Wanda hated to leave. She had worked with most of them for more than eight years.

Trudy, Wanda's closest friend, came by every other day on her way home from work. She would pick up groceries or bring in food for dinner. She sat and talked with Wanda and Kathy, and her good-natured humor was a tonic for both of them. Trudy was the one person Wanda felt she could talk with about anything or everything that worried her.

Kathy began to have trouble concentrating at school. Her mind would wander, and then she would see her mom's face, getting longer and whiter. All these years Kathy had always talked to her mother and told her most everything.

She was Kathy's friend, not just her mother. Kathy always felt proud of her mother. She was pretty, young, and not too strict or old-fashioned, like her best friend Janna's mother.

Lately, Kathy had tried talking more to Janna about what was going on. She told Janna that she kept wishing that she had a horse or that she could ride one. She wanted to feel the freedom of the wind blowing against her as she rode, the freedom to ride away from what was happening. Kathy tried to get out to the fields to see the horses every day. If her mother was home from work, she stayed with her at home after school. Kathy just wanted her to be well, so things could be like they were before. Janna listened to Kathy and then talked about the old saying, "If wishes were horses, then beggars would ride." She said, "Somebody sang a version of it from a few years back that was 'If wishes were horses, then dreamers would ride.'" Janna told Kathy that she probably needed her wishes and dreams now.

Wanda kept getting thinner and weaker. She left work four and a half months after she first saw the doctor. The next week Wanda and Kathy went to the doctor because Wanda was worried about not being able to keep food down, and there was a gnawing pain in her insides, mostly by her ribs. Kathy started out by asking the doctor why he couldn't do anything to help her mother get well. Looking past her, the doctor told Kathy that they just didn't know enough about certain kinds of fast cancers to be able to stop them. He said that he wished that he could have stopped her mother's.

The doctor asked Kathy what kind of help she needed to take care of her mother. Kathy said that she could take care of her, she didn't think she wanted any help. Dr. Johnson said that he thought Kathy and her mom would both need more help, and that he was going to send the hospice people over. Kathy was sure that she could handle it, but Dr. Johnson said hospice would help her mom with her pain, too.

The next day when Kathy got home from school, the hospice nurse, Sue, and the hospice social worker, Elva, were visiting with Wanda. Kathy was quiet and didn't say much when they asked her questions. She didn't want to start crying. After they described the hospice services, Sue said that she would visit Wanda once a week at first, on Friday mornings. She told both Wanda and Kathy that they could call hospice anytime if they needed anything. Before they left, Elva asked Kathy if she could call her once a week or so to see how things were going. Kathy didn't really want her to call, but she said okay just to be polite, and because she knew it would make her mother feel better.

Weeks stretched by, and the days grew longer and the heat was almost at summer levels, even though it was only late April. Kathy thought her mother was growing smaller and she seemed further away. Wanda spent most of her days on the sofa, with the phone nearby. Kathy had been going to school most days, but now she knew that her mother couldn't be alone. It was too hard for her to get up to the bathroom by herself, and sometimes she got mixed up about when she was supposed to take the pain medications.

Elva called and asked Kathy how school was going. Kathy said things were okay, but that she wouldn't be able to go to school. Then Elva asked if she could come out for a visit to help Kathy figure things out. At about six that evening, Elva arrived. She knew that Kathy was a good student at school. She told Kathy that she wanted them all to talk about ways that Kathy could still go to school as much as possible, and have someone to stay and care for her mother. Kathy said that she wanted to be with her mother as much as she could because "I'm the one who knows how to take care of her best." Elva gently said that she thought Kathy could do both, have time together with her mom and attend school as often as she could.

Elva mentioned that Gretta, the nursing assistant, was coming three mornings a week for an hour or so, that might mean that most of those mornings would be covered. Trudy would come by on Mondays, her day off, and stay with Wanda. Sue's nursing visits on Tuesday afternoon and Friday morning would add some coverage, and Elva offered the possibility of a hospice volunteer to help out one morning a week. That way Kathy could go to her classes in the mornings and come home on the afternoons that her mother was alone. Elva suggested, "I know it's not perfect, but it does seem like it will work for the next week or two." Wanda told Kathy how important it was to her that she go to her classes whenever she could. "You know how much I want to spend time with you, Kathy. This way we can do both."

When Trudy came to stay the next Monday, she washed and styled Wanda's long auburn hair. Wanda was exhausted by the effort of doing her hair, so she asked if she could take a short nap and then she wanted to talk with Trudy about Kathy.

Less than an hour later, Wanda awoke from her shallow sleep and looked over at Trudy. "Trudy, I need your help. Would you consider taking in Kathy for me when I'm gone?" Trudy was quiet for a time, and then she asked Wanda, "What do you need me to do?" Wanda told Trudy that she knew Kathy wanted to stay in town, that she felt safe here, with her friends and school, and all that was familiar. "Can you keep her for the school year, and then she can spend the summers with my brother and his family. We can work out whatever legal arrangements sound good to you and Kathy. She's almost thirteen and just about finished with eighth grade. You know she's a good girl and won't give you any trouble. She'll just need somebody to care for her and listen to her."

Trudy considered her life. She was divorced and had no children. At 41, she was sometimes lonely for a family. She'd only been in her present apartment about a year, and it wasn't the greatest. Where would they live? Could she handle Kathy and give her the love that she needed? "Wanda, there's no way on earth that I can replace what you mean to Kathy. I'm smart enough not to even try. Have you asked Kathy what she thinks about your plan?"

"No, because I wanted to talk with you first. If there wasn't a chance, I didn't even want to bring it up. The hospice social worker told me she would help with setting up a foster home or adoption for Kathy when I was ready to talk about it. It feels like it's time to do that now, while I can handle things. If you'll consider it, I'll talk to Kathy in the next day or so."

Trudy agreed, and as she bent down to give Wanda a hug, told her, "You're a good mom to Kathy, and a good friend."

It upset Kathy to tears when her mother brought up the possibility of her staying with Trudy. She didn't want to have to be with anyone besides her mother. For the last weeks Kathy had worried every day about where she would live and who would take care of her. And, she didn't want to leave Greenville. Maybe it was just any other small Southern town of 20,000 people, but it was home. Kathy thought about the horses and leaving the place she had always lived. It was just too much. So, she agreed to the meeting to talk about living with Trudy.

Wanda couldn't imagine anything more heartbreaking about this whole situation than to talk about who would care for her daughter after she was gone. Dying wouldn't be so bad if it didn't mean leaving the people that you loved. She wanted to see Kathy grow up and marry, and she would have liked to have been able to be a grandmother. Most of all, she would have liked to see Kathy become a woman so they could discover different ways of being mother and daughter together.

It was Wednesday evening when Elva, the hospice social worker, met with Wanda, Kathy, and Trudy. She had already spoken with the people at Child Protective Services about their regulations and ways to proceed. Kathy could be placed with Trudy as a permanent foster home, and Wanda's brother would become Kathy's legal guardian. When they talked, Kathy was reserved, finally saying that she did want to live with Trudy. "But is it possible that we could live in this house?"

Trudy said that she would be willing to consider the possibility, and asked Kathy if they could look around at some places later on before they decided for sure. "My place won't work since it's only a one bedroom. I'm not happy with it anyway, and we have some time to decide. I'll come stay with you here whenever you and your mother feel it's right. You won't have to be alone."

Kathy turned 13 the second week in May. Trudy picked up the gift that Wanda wanted to give to Kathy, a necklace with a gold horse charm. The surprise gift was from Trudy: three horseback-riding lessons at the local ranch. Even though she tried not to, Kathy cried. She had dreaded this birthday, but it was one she would always remember.

Violet, Wanda's friend, called the next week and told Wanda that she had arranged for Twila Starr to come out to the house on Thursday afternoon. Wanda was pleased, but she wasn't sure that she wanted to take any more herbs. "Just let her come and talk to you and do her healing touch. It can't hurt," Violet persisted. Kathy was already home from school when Twila arrived after four. She brought with her that peaceful air that Wanda had remembered. Before she did the healing touch, they talked. Wanda began, "I didn't really expect to be cured, but I had hoped that I could have more time."

Twila asked, "Has the time that you've had been good, and did you spend it the way that you wanted?"

"Yes," Wanda admitted, "except for the weakness. But I worked a month longer than the doctor expected that I could, and Kathy and I have had some sweet times."

"Then is there anything else that you want to look at now?"

Wanda hesitated, then began, "I don't know what I believe happens when you die. Of course, we go to church, and I believe in heaven, but I wonder how the actual dying will be."

Twila responded, "Do you have any ideas about it, or any experiences that would help you with this?"

"Well, my daddy died in the hospital when I was nine, and I didn't get to see him till after he was gone. My mother died of a heart attack, so it was fast, and again I only saw her at the funeral home." Wanda pulled up her strength. "I never told you, but when you laid your hands on my head, I experienced a strange purple circle of light with a golden center and a green shiny edge around it. It moved in and out and changed some, but I always felt like it was calling to me. The only way I can describe it is serene, and refreshing, like you feel just when you get out of the bath." Kathy sat by and listened intently to what her mother was saying.

Twila looked from mother to daughter and then said, "What you describe was a different state of consciousness that some people find when they meditate or pray. It may offer you some clues about what dying is like. Dying is a mystery, and we just don't really know. I have seen several people die, and it was not frightening, only quiet, a passing away to another place, like you talked about. Maybe it isn't as important to think about what will happen when you die. Kathy will be here, and the people from hospice too, I'm sure. The most important thing now is to live the best and most loving ways possible and that will prepare you for what's ahead. That's true for you, too, Kathy. I don't understand all that happens with death, and I wish this wasn't your time so soon. You have a beautiful spirit, Wanda. Just trust the love that is around you, both of you." With that, the three were silent and Twila laid her hands first on Wanda's ribs, and then on her head. Then, she went over to Kathy and asked if she could touch her head as well. Kathy felt soothed by her touch. Twila hugged both Wanda and Kathy and left.

On Sue's regular visit that Friday, Wanda brought up Twila Starr's visit. She had never mentioned to any of the hospice people that she had seen the healer. Sue listened and then said, "She sounds like a remarkable woman. What she did with you certainly seems like a kind of healing. It didn't heal your cancer, but it strengthened you and brought healing to your heart and spirit. From what you've told me, it gave you some measure of hope, and seems to have been a positive experience for you, and for Kathy, too. Twila was right about dying. It's not that scary when it's actually happening. It's thinking about it ahead of time that's hard. Remember, Wanda, you won't be alone. I've told both you and Kathy that you can call hospice any time that you need us, and one of the nurses will be here. We'll be here with you both."

As the days passed, Wanda's weakness grew, and she was able to eat very little. For the past few weeks she'd only been drinking liquid protein supplements. Eventually, Wanda moved back to her bedroom, where hospice had delivered a hospital bed and a bedside commode. Kathy never went to school during those last three weeks. She stayed by her mother and cared for her "better than anyone else could."

On the third of June, Wanda died. Kathy and the hospice nurse were with her. There were three or four hours earlier in the day when she was very restless, but Sue got some medication that Dr. Johnson ordered and it calmed Wanda down shortly after. Then she began to drift away, even though Kathy still talked to her and played her favorite music in the room. When Wanda was gone, Kathy cried a long time, and lay on the bed next to her and cuddled with her, just as she had done so often these last weeks. Then, Kathy picked out a purple dress for her mother to wear. She knew this was real, she just wanted it all to be a dream. She wanted to have her mother back.

Kathy didn't remember much about the funeral. The pastor said some very kind things about her mother, and there were over a hundred people there. Kathy sat next to Trudy and her Uncle Pete, and Janna was in the pew behind them. There was food at Violet's after. Kathy didn't like having so many strange people hugging her. She wanted to run away and be by herself. Later, Janna said they would go out to the horses and that would help. Kathy was glad it was summer and she would not have to go to school. Because of all the decisions about where to live with Trudy, Kathy wasn't going out to her Uncle Pete's until July sometime. He was being very understanding, and Kathy liked him. It would be nice to be with her cousins for a while.

Kathy didn't want to think too much right now. She just wanted to get through today and to try to stay close to her mother in her thoughts. One night, Kathy saw her mother in her dream, and she smiled and told Kathy that she was all right. She said, "I'll always be near you and with you, Kathy." The dream stayed with Kathy, like a warm glow inside. She wanted to keep it close. She knew it was a special gift from her mother.

> *Hold on to what is good*
> *even if it is*
> *a handful of earth.*
> *Hold on to what you believe*
> *even if it is*
> *a tree which stands by itself.*
> *Hold on to what you must do*
> *even if it is*
> *a long way from here.*
> *Hold on to life even when*
> *it is easier letting go.*
> *Hold on to my hand even when*
> *I have gone away from you.*
>
> —NANCY WOOD
> *MANY WINTERS*

CAREGIVING REALITIES
A Small Family

One of the major changes experienced in our culture this century is the dispersion and shrinking of the family. Families in North America are smaller, with fewer children and perhaps only one parent living in the home. Fewer families have relatives that they can count on within a fifty-mile distance. The proximity and availability of family members to young widows with children has been found to be a major determinant of the outcome of bereavement.[1] Many families, like Wanda and Kathy, do not have blood relatives nearby. In addition to the adaptations to illness that are necessary, families must search for the support that they need from within their circle of friends and the resources available close by.

Caregiver Shortage

It is not an overstatement to say that there is a serious shortage of caregivers in our country. Not only are families smaller, but both partners are typically employed outside the home. Or, in the case of the elderly, the caregiving spouse may also be frail and is not able to take on the full weight of caregiving. And families with only one parent are at a distinct disadvantage. Caregiving responsibilities must then fall to the children in the home. The burdens that children and adolescents face as caregivers are complex. Children like Kathy feel fearful, isolated, and alone, and sometimes overwhelmed in their caregiving role. They can also have a strong sense of loyalty and duty to care for their ill parent.[2]

Children and Adolescents as Caregivers

Grief typically involves feelings of a loss of innocence and illusions, of growing older because of the experience. This reality can be intensified when the child is caring for a dying parent and feels confounded by the magnitude of the tasks. There can also be a sense of failure at the parent's death. It is an especially painful reversal of traditional roles, when the caregiving parent must be cared for by the child. .

Adolescents and children who become caregivers for a seriously ill and dying parent also lose the role of being the child or adolescent. The demands of caregiving that mean time away from school rob adolescents and children of the means to meet their friendship and peer needs.

Caregiving is particularly difficult for adolescents who are struggling with the process of separation from the parent or family. Adolescents are faced with rapidly changing emotions and responses, and the familiar shadow of ambivalence. The grieving teen can feel burdened by extra measures of guilt and resentment in an already difficult time. Grieving teens and children find it helpful to have consistent adults available for nurturing and to buffer the demands and distress of the caregiving situation.

New Caregiving Approaches

Typically, there is a main person providing care for the one who is ill, with the backup and assistance of others. Because the burdens of caregiving can be so great, and because not everyone has an available caregiver, alternative ways need to be considered. In a recent book, *Share the Care*, Caposella and Warnock discuss ways to organize a group to provide care for someone who is seriously ill.[3] Speaking from their own experience as part of a caregiving group, they outline the ways to start a group, share caregiving responsibilities, and keep the group going. Their discussion also focuses on the costs and rewards of caregiving. The collective approach they describe is one possible solution to the critical need for caregivers.

The Power of Denial

It is easy to wonder why Wanda waited before seeking medical help. She "believed it would go away." Denial is an attractive and powerful force in adapting to painful realities. A classic defense mechanism, it helps us keep reality at bay, at least for a while. In truth, all human beings use some measure of denial just to get through the day-to-day threats life poses. In his

1973 Pulitzer Prize–winning book *The Denial of Death*, Ernest Becker explores many of the ways, as individuals and as members of a society, we try to insulate ourselves from the awareness and fears of the reality of personal death.[4]

Newspapers are laden with accounts of natural disasters, traffic fatalities, and other death-related tragedies that we glance at sideways. We can feel concern for others affected by the tragedies, but somehow we are left with a sense of relief and an illusion of safety.

Denial can serve a useful purpose in that it buys us time to absorb the reality and to consider other ways of responding. Initially, avoidance, which is the major dynamic involved in denial, is a natural attempt to keep reality at arm's length. In the short run, it also allows us to stay functional and engaged with our day-to-day lives and their requirements. There is an almost instinctive response to deny painful possibilities. Paraphrasing Thornton Wilder in his provocative novel about random death, *The Bridge of San Luis Rey*, denial springs eternal in the human breast.

Denial can be debilitating and dangerous. If denial is the only major defense, and if it is perpetuated across time, it severely limits our coping abilities. Ongoing denial becomes an extreme response that internally involves the message "I can't deal with this, so I'll just go on and act as if it's not there." That message implies a low level of confidence in one's abilities to handle difficult situations, like a life-threatening illness. While no one ever feels able to cope with painful potentials, the ability to look at the face of reality is essential. Only that vision will inform us about our possible reactions and responses.

Denial Versus Hope

Does sustained denial keep us in a state of anesthesia that is a barrier against feeling life in its harsh expressions? Or, if we look at the realities of our circumstances, with all of their encroaching difficulty, does that mean that we give up hope and become mired in our situation? We deny initially to protect ourselves against what seems like an overwhelming and unacceptable reality because we are afraid and do not want to deal with it. In our attempt to resist an unwelcome change in our world, we seek to maintain equilibrium and forestall, a negative future. Adaptation to difficult circumstances involves problem-solving and coping that address the situation directly. Only then can we balance the stresses and sustain feelings of competency.

Hopes and Fears

Perhaps one of our greatest fears related to serious illness is that of losing hope. Hopelessness is the state where we are unable to tolerate our situation. All reasons for continuing are gone, all attachment to others withdrawn. Life in this condition is unlivable. Feelings of helplessness seem inevitably intertwined with those of hopelessness.

Just as fear and hope are interconnected, hope can come out of despair. The classic image of transcending hopelessness is of the phoenix rising from the ashes. We typically associate hope with some *reason* that gives birth or rebirth to it. Even when the diagnosis of a life-threatening illness is made, there are still tangible reasons for hope that typically exist. These specific hopes related to a life-threatening illness could be seen as part of the progressive attempt to reconcile with changing, uncontrollable circumstances:

- Hope for a cure
- Hope for good treatment outcomes
- Hope for more time
- Hope for meaningful, loving time
- Hope for the strength to bear things well
- Hope for a death consistent with one's own ways and style
- Hope for a continuation of life after death
- Hope for reunion with deceased loved ones.

> *What you have to fight is hopelessness—even under torment, despite whatever calamities, however bleak the outlook. Hope is the keystone; faith and courage-with-pride are the two pillars on which it rests.*
>
> —EDWIN SHNEIDMAN

Hospice and Hope

While these hopes evolve during the progression of a terminal illness, hospice offers people who are dying possibilities to explore or fulfill many of them. It is not unusual for physicians to delay in making the referral to a hospice program because they believe it would be too disheartening for the person to realize that there was limited time. Dr. Johnson presented hospice as a way to help both Wanda and Kathy. The trusted family physician engenders confidence in the hospice program by the encouraging, positive manner in which the services are presented.

Truthfully, no one welcomes being told that a referral to hospice is indicated. Some hospices are expanding their range of services to include preterminal "bridge" programs to offer care to families prior to the last weeks of life. The belief is that hospice services could offer valuable support to families in advance of the last two months of life. Other reasons to offer preterminal care is that it may, at least in part, diminish some of the death stigma associated with hospice and also maximize referrals. Families show little reluctance and, typically, great relief once they begin receiving hospice care and supportive services.

Finally, in looking at Wanda's story, we can see that she initially used denial to avoid what was certainly a devastating diagnosis. Wanda faced her situation once the diagnosis was made and surgery had taken place. She focused her energies on maintaining her relationships with her daughter, Kathy, and her friends and coworkers. When people who are dying relate to people who are able to acknowledge that death is imminent, denial stops.[5] Hospice can play an important role in creating opportunities for both the person who is dying and the family members to move past denial to a sense of calm strength around a reality that can be faced together.

> *Hope is like the sun, which as we journey toward it, casts the shadow of our burden behind us.*
>
> —SAMUEL SMILES

Chapter Eight

WAITING TO LIVE
A Couple's Retirement Dream Changes

Whenever your life ends, it is all there. The advantage of living is not measured by length, but by use; some men have lived long, and lived little; attend to it while you are in it. It lies in your will, not in the number of years, for you to have lived enough.

—Michel Eyquem de Montaigne

Larry Haute is 66 years old and his wife, Maureen, is 63; they have been married for thirty-nine years. Both Larry and Maureen are retired, he from a major film and photographic supply company where he was a shift supervisor for almost ten years prior to his retirement after thirty-three years with the company. Maureen was a part-time bookkeeper for a small family-owned tire store. Larry and Maureen have two children, Gene and Barbara. Both children are married, have their own children, and live out-of-state. As a result of the distances involved and the pressures of raising their own families, Gene and Barbara are not close to Larry and Maureen, but do try to stay in routine contact with monthly telephone calls and yearly holiday visits. They describe themselves as a typical American family.

With their savings and Larry's pension, the Hautes were looking forward to a comfortable retirement. They made plans to visit Europe, and were thinking about purchasing a motor-home for touring the United States during the next several years. Prior to leaving for Europe, Larry decided to have a routine physical exam, as his last exam had been a company-sponsored one more than two years ago.

As part of the physical examination, Larry's doctor performed a routine prostate-specific antigen (PSA) test. Larry mentioned to Dr. Montgomery that lately he had been getting up several times during the night to urinate, and that his hips had been bothering him. Larry told his doctor that he'd passed both problems off as the result of getting older. Dr. Montgomery responded that he was concerned, because such symptoms could indicate problems of the prostate. Dr. Montgomery said he would contact him as soon as the PSA test results were available. The following week, Dr. Montgomery called Larry and told him that his PSA was extremely elevated. A second PSA test confirmed the results of the first and Dr. Montgomery referred Larry to Dr. Arori, a urologist in the same practice.

The results of a biopsy and further tests were later reported to Larry—he had cancer of the prostate. Dr. Arori scheduled Larry to have a bone scan and a CT scan X ray. Three weeks after his initial exam, Larry learned that the cancer had metastasized to his bones. A third PSA showed even higher levels than the original results. Larry and Maureen were faced with several treatment options. They rejected a radical prostatectomy in favor of radiation therapy, although the bony metastasis had created a sense of foreboding. Over the course of the next year Larry was treated first with radiation therapy. During this seven-week period Larry received radiation treatments five days per week.

Following radiation therapy, Larry's PSA levels remained elevated and additional tests confirmed the presence of continued metastatic disease. The next therapy to be offered was a form of chemotherapy using hormones. Unfortunately, Larry's prognosis worsened. Dr. Arori and Dr. Montgomery told him and Maureen that it was unlikely that he would live more than six months. Larry was growing weaker, the result of the cancer and the treatments. He was also in pain, which was becoming more difficult to suppress. Maureen needed help to be able to care for Larry. Dr. Montgomery suggested that he make a referral to the community hospice program. Larry and Maureen reluctantly agreed. Larry had not established an advance directive, but he knew that he did not want to spend the last weeks of his life in a hospital. Maureen felt that with help she would be able to manage the care Larry would need.

At first, Larry and Maureen felt relieved by the hospice's involvement. Larry's pain was controlled adequately for the first time in months; he was awake much of the day, slept during the night, and was able to engage others in conversation. He and Maureen were able to talk and Maureen was able to spend some time in her garden. Their children came for a visit, and Maureen went away for the weekend while the hospice program provided inpatient respite care in a local nursing home.

Still, it was a sad home. Although it made her furious at herself, Maureen could not help but feel anger at Larry for dying, and bitterness about how her life had turned. This was supposed to be a time of promise and reward for years of hard work. Instead, Maureen faced the even harder work of caring for Larry's physical needs. Both Larry and Maureen had seen their lives as just beginning; so many things had been put on hold while they made it through the days, which turned to months and then into years. When they were retired, they would begin to live. Now, Maureen knew that soon she would be alone.

To their credit, and with the help of the hospice team, Larry and Maureen began to see the value of their lives. They began to focus on their love for each other and their family and slowly Maureen became less bitter about Larry's impending death. Still, they were both aware that while hospice care could help them pack more life into the remaining days they had together, they could never go back and put more life in the days they had already lived.

With Larry becoming weaker, it was already becoming more difficult to care for him. The hospice was visiting more often, with the nurse coming several times per week and the nursing assistants four times each week. Dr. Montgomery felt the hospice physician would be better able to care for Larry, so the hospice's medical director, Dr. Connie Barrett, became Larry's attending physician and she came by the house about every ten days. Dr. Barrett also spoke with Larry and Maureen by phone as often as they felt necessary. Their daughter, Barbara, came to help for a week, and it appeared that the family would maintain its promise to Larry to keep him at home.

It was a mild summer morning and Maureen was up early, working in her garden while Larry slept. Maureen felt odd that morning as she pruned her roses. She thought she was just more tired than usual, but she quickly began to feel worse and barely managed to get to the phone. Maureen was confused, she didn't know what to do so she called Dr. Barrett, who recognized that Maureen was in trouble and immediately called for an ambulance.

Maureen had suffered what her doctor later described to her as a "mild stroke." She was in no current danger, and she was out of the hospital in four days. She would receive rehabilitation therapy from the local home-health agency. Barbara again moved into the house, but this time to help care for her mother. During Maureen's hospitalization, Larry was transferred to the hospice's inpatient unit. Larry could stay in the inpatient unit for several more days; however, the hospice unit was intended to be for brief admissions for acute needs, including a crisis. Maureen visited Larry as soon as she was able, and she was delighted to see that even though the nurses and aides were different, Larry's regular nurse came to visit, and nothing had changed as far as the goals of the care he was receiving.

Again, Larry and Maureen were faced with decisions. Larry was not in need of acute inpatient care, but Maureen was no longer strong enough to care for Larry at home, and Barbara would soon have to return home to care for her own children. Another option was needed.

Hospice suggested placing Larry in their residential program. The Hautes would have to pay for the room-and-board portion of the care, but Medicare would continue to pay for all hospice services. Larry and Maureen agreed that living in the hospice residence would be best for Larry and for everyone. Several days later, Larry moved into the Hospice House.

Once more, Larry's caregivers changed; however, the plan of care that had been developed when Larry first entered the hospice program remained the same. During the three weeks that Larry stayed in the residential program, the goal remained pain- and symptom-control. As he became weaker, Larry stopped eating, and there were no attempts to start to force food by tube feedings. Larry continued to drink a little water, but he and Maureen had decided against any artificial hydration. Maureen continued to live at home, and would visit Larry every day. She occasionally stayed overnight in Larry's room.

Larry died late on a Wednesday night in September, after Maureen had gone home. Larry's funeral was small: his family, a few neighbors, some of his coworkers, and several members of the hospice staff. As Maureen had told the hospice social worker, there hadn't been much time for friends— it was something they'd been looking forward to after they retired. Maureen attends the hospice's bereavement support group now, and is beginning to make new friends. She has been making plans to visit Europe next summer.

Hospice Inpatient Care

Almost 90 percent of all hospice care days are spent in the patient's home. Certainly, over the years, the definition of what we consider home has changed dramatically. Two decades ago, "home" would have been defined as a two-story colonial in the suburbs or perhaps an apartment downtown. Today, hospice patients live in their personal residence, but also in congregate living facilities, some owned and operated by hospices and often referred to as a hospice residence. Others live in nursing homes and still others are technically homeless. Hospice programs provide services in all of these "homes."

 - Many times, hospice facilities are referred to as "inpatient units," which is not technically correct, because—as in Larry's case—a facility can also identify a residential program. Hospice inpatient care is primarily acute care provided in a facility. Such care usually involves management of pain and symptoms that cannot be cared for adequately in the patient's home. Occasionally, inpatient care will also include a surgical procedure. Additionally, inpatient care is available to a patient whose caregiver experiences a crisis and is unable to continue to provide care. Maureen's stroke is a good example.

Most inpatient stays are of a short duration, fewer than ten days. Inpatient hospice care is a covered service under the Medicare/Medicaid Hospice Benefit and most commercial insurers. While some hospices own and operate an inpatient facility, other hospices lease space from an existing hospital or nursing home and then care for patients using their own staff. However, the overwhelming number of hospices provide inpatient care by contracting with a hospital or nursing facility to provide such care under the supervision of the patient's individual plan of care. As noted in chapter 1, this care plan guides the work of the interdisciplinary team. Perhaps more importantly, this plan of care frames the care that is provided across all possible settings.

Respite Care

The basis for the great successes of hospice care is the extraordinary strength of the patients' caregivers. And, while the rewards to the patient and the caregiver can be enormous, caring for a spouse or loved one in your home is hard work. Even with the talents of the hospice team to support the efforts of the caregiver and the family, physical and emotional exhaustion can challenge the commitment of the most resolute caregiver. To assist caregivers facing this challenge, hospice programs provide a respite service so that family caregivers can have a few days off, get a good night's sleep, or simply take a walk or go shopping.

Some respite care is provided in the patient's home by volunteers and staff, from a few hours up to several days. In some cases, the patient is cared for in a facility (most often a skilled-nursing facility) where the hospice has a specific contract for these services. The Medicare/Medicaid Hospice Benefit provides a specific payment to hospices for the provision of respite care in a facility, and expects that respite care provided in the patient's home will be made available on an intermittent basis as part of the general home-care payment.

Alternatives Within Hospice Care

As the population ages, hospices are increasingly serving patients whose spouse or significant other is too frail to care for a dying person in their home. There are also increasing numbers of people who live alone and are dying. In the past, these people would have found themselves in a revolving-door situation with hospital admissions: discharged to their homes with little or no care or support from the outside until they deteriorated to the point of needing to be admitted to the hospital again. The cycle would repeat until their last admission to the hospital. Increasingly, however, people who do not have a caregiver in their home are finding their way into hospice programs and hospice programs are facing the challenge of caring for them.

Most dying people who live in nursing homes can receive their hospice care from a community hospice program contracted by the nursing home to provide such services.

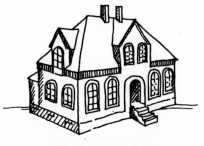

Hospice Residence
Residential Facility

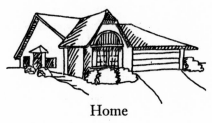

Home

Where
Hospice Care
Takes Place

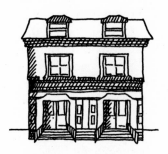

Nursing Home
Hospice Unit/Wing

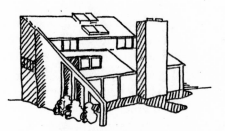

Hospital/Hospice
Inpatient Unit

Nursing visits, consultation with the nursing home staff, and a plan of care are all part of hospice services to nursing home residents.

Hospice also provides what is sometimes called the "substitute caregiver program." Not every hospice program offers this service, but it is an arrangement where a paid caregiver (or occasionally a volunteer) is hired to provide virtually around-the-clock assistance to the person who is dying. Such services could include bathing, feeding, grooming, assistance with medication (if permitted by law), and transportation.

Unfortunately, most payment sources do not pay for these services, so the caregiver receives wages directly from the patient and family. This can be quite expensive over a period of weeks and months. In some states, Medicaid pays for such services under certain conditions.

A small number of hospice programs have begun to institute day-care programs. These programs are designed to provide a setting for the dying person to come to during the day, returning to their own home at night. Such services are invaluable to the spouse who could not cope with caregiver responsibility on a full-time basis, but who is able to serve adequately in this capacity when provided relief from some of the caregiving burden. Few insurance programs cover the cost of day-care services so these costs are usually borne by the patient and family. Some hospices have been able to reduce the costs of day care through philanthropic support. The cost of day care is almost always less than full-time care in a hospice residence or nursing home.

An emerging focus of care that responds to the needs of those who cannot be kept in their own homes is the increasing number of hospices that are establishing residential programs. Although many would refer to hospice care provided in the nursing home or even care provided in congregate living facilities as residential care, residential hospice care is more frequently coming to mean hospice care provided in a facility—most often one owned by the hospice program.

Most hospice residential facilities are quite small, often

occupying a house that has been retrofitted to meet the needs of the patients and professional caregivers. A small number of residential programs are housed in special hospice facilities that also provide acute inpatient care. These facilities are almost always associated with large hospices, and are usually quite large themselves.

A residential program and inpatient hospice care differ even if provided in the same facility. Inpatient care usually requires a significant medical need that cannot be addressed in the patient's home. Residential care is provided to patients who simply cannot be kept safely in their own home.

Most hospice residential programs report being fully occupied most of the time, so in many communities there can be a waiting list for patients wanting to use the hospice residential facility. The average stay in a residential hospice facility is around thirty days, and currently there is little third-party insurance coverage for the residential care. Occasionally some managed care companies do cover this type of service as an alternative to hospitalization. Additionally, hospice programs often charge for residential care on a sliding-scale fee basis. Medicare, as well as Medicaid and commercial insurers, will pay hospices a routine home-care rate for each day of hospice care delivered in a residential facility.

These emerging forms of hospice care expand the ability of hospices to serve greater numbers of people in their communities. Although such services are still new and not widely available across the country, many hospices are evaluating the possibility of adding such services, and we can expect much broader availability in the near future.

Chapter Nine

IT DOESN'T SEEM LIKE SUCH A LONG TIME NOW

Two Families Face the End Together

"Long-term survivor." The descriptor has connotations of a tenacious dance with the end of life, but at some time in the future. "Long-term survivor" also means that many people are counting on you to be there.

Gregg returned home from his monthly appointment—not an appointment, really, more like a visit, since this routine visit had gone on long enough to be considered a professional relationship that had turned into a friendship. Perhaps that is what the practice of medicine should really be, and what it was at one time.

It had been nine years last month. So why did this visit with Alex—Dr. Alex Martin—have to be so different. What happened? Why now? Gregg was used to the routine, to the tests, to the numbers, nothing had changed in such a long time, it had just become part of everyday life, a good life, some would even call it fortunate. But today's visit called for a cab home, instead of the subway. It called for stopping by the corner vendor for a hot dog. It called for a walk in the park.

Quiet time has always been important to Gregg, but today it is both affirming and disturbing. Calm on the outside and shaking on the inside, he wandered from the bridge to the benches around the pond. This has always been a favorite spot for Gregg to come to think, to reflect, and to wonder, so the path was familiar, comfortable, and even reassuring.

He spoke to people on the path as usual, just a "hi" or "hello" or "how are you," but the park was friendly and it was almost the standard. He hoped no one asked how he was today; he wasn't sure he could say anything. Gregg noticed lots of people in the park this afternoon. Most of the time when he stopped it was on the way home, not in the middle of the day. It was nice to see it more crowded in the middle of the day. Mothers and children in the park—it made for nice surroundings while he was trying not to think. Sitting quietly on the park bench, Gregg remembered those weekends from his childhood when his mother and dad and sister would feed the ducks at the park, and swing and slide for hours on the "twisted" slide. What he wouldn't give for those same safe and warm feelings now.

Shaken back into the present by a ball that landed at his feet, Gregg knew the person who shared his life would soon be asking how his visit was with Dr. Martin. Since his response to this question had been the same for so long, it would be harder now to tell Anthony about these drastic changes in his health status. "The status of his disease"—it almost sounds like something separate from who you are and how you are. The disease has now progressed. Progress in almost every other sense of the word is a positive thing, but certainly not in this instance.

Gregg wasn't feeling all that bad, or perhaps he just wasn't letting himself realize or assimilate those feelings into his daily living. He knew things had changed, that he had been sick more often—sometimes quietly, but more often. He was doing more work at home, and getting less done on research projects than he wanted to acknowledge. As Anthony reminded him on a regular basis, Gregg was much more fortunate than most all of their friends dealing with this disease, as he held a position as a college professor that included a certain degree of flexibility. He had the freedom to work intensely when he felt well and take the time necessary to cope with his illness when he was sick. He knew he was fortunate in many, many ways. He had access to all the new drugs. But right now he didn't feel very fortunate. In fact, he felt like the ball that landed at his feet had hit him in the stomach. He was trying to catch his breath and felt cramping at the same time. He would need to find the restroom soon.

Putting the key in the lock of their apartment, Gregg still wasn't sure what he would say to Anthony. Maybe Anthony already knew more than Gregg thought. They had stopped focusing on AIDS since it had been such a part of their lives for so long now, and everyone who was on protease inhibitors (PIs) was doing great. Why weren't they working for him? Anthony was in the kitchen cooking dinner. "Pasta with veggies, almost ready" resonated from the kitchen when Gregg shut and turned the locks on the door. Safe, home, secure—everything would be fine.

As Anthony looked at Gregg, he didn't need to ask how his visit with Alex had been; the tears quietly streaming down Gregg's face told him. Anthony opened his strong arms wide to offer Gregg the comforting hug and embrace he so desperately needed. Other than the CD playing in the living room, it was intensely quiet, as if the tears from both men said everything, for now.

It's amazing how easy, perhaps too easy, it is to compartmentalize thoughts and feelings. Neither man brought up the doctor's visit all through dinner, or as they discussed the rest of the day's activities. They put a movie in the VCR: *Auntie Mame* was the selection of the evening. Glistening humor without the need for intense thinking could be a very good thing. "Books are so decorative," was about as deep as either wanted to take the evening entertainment.

Tomorrow was Saturday, time for sleeping late, regrouping, lunch out, perhaps at the Garden Room, if the wait in line could be tolerated, and conversation . . . the conversation. Sleep was not easy for either of them. After tossing and turning, Anthony heard the tub filling; it was only nine o'clock, early for a weekend day. Anthony decided to read for a while, giving Gregg the quiet time he knew he needed to immerse himself in the tub. Anthony read and dozed off and on for the next hour, although it seemed like several hours, before Gregg came back into the bedroom to get dressed. They made distant small talk. The realization crossed Anthony's mind that Gregg had gotten much thinner during this past few weeks. Although he knew it wasn't drastic, it just seemed so much more when he concentrated on what was happening.

It was raining out. How appropriate. Gregg felt like he was being poured on, so at least real rain would be symbolic, if nothing else. As Anthony showered and dressed, Gregg thought about how much he and Anthony had been involved in fighting this disease, the books they had read, the blocks they had marched, the buddies they cared for, and the hours they volunteered. And in all this time, how could they have almost, if not totally, avoided the conversations about the end of life? After starting PIs, with such high expectations, this was like hearing the diagnosis all over again.

Until now, it seemed to always be about the fight, the drugs, the opportunistic infections (OIs) of the month, the family, the other family, and the memorial service. The dialogue for this part of the conversation was new. Others had to have had it. Did they just miss it? Gregg had a history of rehearsing dialogue in his head, priding himself on being quite articulate, even confident in participating in difficult, important, yet delicate conversations. Now he felt like a spectator, wondering if he had missed this whole part, or perhaps he just didn't want to think about it, and that was why nothing was coming to him. Nothing. None of his thoughts were coming together, or even felt rational for that matter. Anthony did a little soft-shoe in the bedroom to get Gregg's attention; it worked, it always worked, and brought a smile to his face at the same time.

Gregg's diagnosis of HIV early in the partnership had shaken the security of the relationship once. He was afraid this most recent change might shake it again. He knew better in his heart, but he couldn't help thinking about everything to come. This was clearly going to involve issues never before addressed or even discussed. Their friends called it new territory, and it scared Gregg that it was even defined.

The morning of shopping had been great, and late lunch at Saks superb. There was something about lunch in a department store that took Gregg back to his childhood, when lunch with his grandmother in the department store tearoom was very special. He missed her. She had been gone for years, but he missed her. Gregg knew that she recognized the things in him that were different and she approved. He drew on that approval a great deal as he was growing up, since there were lots of other folks who didn't offer that same level of understanding.

After lunch, Gregg asked Anthony if they could make one additional stop. Gregg's time out was catching up with him quickly. Gregg headed to the fifth floor, to the silver department, with Anthony asking him what it was that he was looking for that he didn't already have. The store didn't have what he wanted, so Gregg ordered one sterling silver demitasse spoon in Grand Baroque. He then explained to Anthony that when he was little he went with his grandmother to the department store whenever he visited, and she would buy one piece of sterling at a time. It was such a big event, because each spoon cost more than ten dollars. Anthony knew Gregg had a large set of sterling. They used it often, especially when guests were over. He knew it was especially important to Gregg, but until today he didn't have the story to connect to the value. Gregg told Anthony that he still had only eleven demitasse spoons and he needed one more to complete the set, and even at almost one hundred dollars for that tiny little spoon, he needed to be sure the set was complete.

Anthony took Gregg's hand, something they never did in public, to offer him support and strength as he headed toward the escalator. Anthony did his best to keep himself focused and calm, but he wasn't sure how long he could maintain this level of presence with so many things running through his mind.

Gregg wanted to walk a couple of blocks before catching a cab, just to get some air. But two blocks became one, and not quite one at that, and Anthony hailed a cab to take them back home.

Gregg broke down almost immediately after entering the foyer. Anthony held him and helped him get to the sofa in the living room. It hit both of them at the same time that these changes that were occurring were life-changing events, not just another battle in the aggressive fight they had been waging for so many years. It was no longer just about an opportunistic infection, it was about everything. They were at the point of making decisions.

Gregg had rehearsed the very end of his life in his mind from the first time he received his diagnosis. He would be in charge, and it would be scripted as if it were a theater performance. Anthony would direct, and the scores of players would play their parts, although a whole lot of the players were no longer available to be on the stage. And he would have his family with him. It would make them realize the city was not a place to be afraid of, but a place to be enjoyed. But it had become clear to him over the past few months that this disease called AIDS did the directing, that the stage was complex and the players uncertain, and that his family didn't even know he was sick. How were they going to begin to know how to play their parts?

Gregg was a very fortunate person living with AIDS (although he hated the PLWA acronym) in that he didn't look sick, just thinner—although now, perhaps, that was not to his benefit, since it was so hard for Anthony, and others, to realize he was so very sick. It was even hard for his doctors and nurses, even with repeated hospital visits for infections, to process how sick he was. But for Gregg it was the most gracious of God's gifts, perhaps the only one he would consider gracious, during this entire trip with HIV and AIDS, that he at least never appeared sick to the majority of his family and friends.

It was so hard to begin, but once Gregg got started, he

and Anthony talked for hours. They discussed Alex's reports, questions, and recommendations. Alex had told Gregg, nearly a year ago, that the time would come when he would need to make a decision about how aggressively he wanted to fight to extend his life, versus an aggressive protocol to provide for quality of life at the end of life. Now this conflict was real and although he knew what he wanted to do, he wasn't sure what others would expect of him and, in turn, what that would allow him to do.

That conversation with Alex had floated in and out of Gregg's mind for the past several months. Gregg had been an involved patient from the very beginning, reading, studying, and participating in his own care. He had served as a buddy, as a caregiver for several friends; he knew about death. And although Gregg thought he was ready to transition his plan of care to focus on the ways he wanted to spend his days, he wasn't sure anyone else was at that same place. His buddies would think he was giving up, Anthony would think he wasn't fighting hard enough to stay with him. Everyone knows that if you just fight hard enough you can beat this disease; he had beat it so many times before.

Anthony made sure Gregg knew he would support him in whatever his decisions were, and be there, and love him, even if it was hard. It was only seven o'clock in the evening, but Gregg went to sleep and didn't wake up until after nine the next morning, a sleep he clearly needed. It was quiet time Anthony needed as well. Sleep came with difficulty for the one who had just agreed to be strong and brave.

Alex had told Gregg that he worked with several hospice programs that provided comprehensive care for many of his other patients with AIDS. Two of the hospices even had specialized AIDS-care programs, with staff who were very knowledgeable and experienced in caring for individuals with AIDS.

Anthony made three calls, just to get some basic information for Gregg, although it seemed Gregg had the basic information, and it was Anthony who really needed to be reassured as to what hospice care was all about. Anthony had, like Gregg, served as a buddy, a supportive volunteer similar to a hospice volunteer, for over three years. Though he already had quite a bit of information, he realized he clearly had some misconceptions about hospice care.

First, Gregg's care would be provided in their apartment, unless there was a clear need for being in the hospital or somewhere else. Second, the volunteer buddies Gregg and Anthony already knew could work with the hospice staff to provide care. Gregg's insurance, which had been great to date, included a hospice benefit. Anthony felt fine with his conversations with all three programs. One program was actually in close proximity to their neighborhood, so he made an appointment for two staff members to come over to their home to meet with both of them.

Prior to the hospice staff arriving, Anthony called Alex from his office just to reassure himself that what they were doing was appropriate. Anthony was hoping in the back of his mind that Alex would say maybe they should put off this meeting, that maybe it wasn't time yet. He didn't. All Alex did was to reassure Anthony that they did have some decisions and choices to make and that this was probably the time for it to happen. No, as he told Gregg, he couldn't make finite declarations about time. If only he could; it was clear things had changed and were progressive at this point.

The meeting with the hospice staff had been set for four o'clock in the afternoon. Anthony left the office early and was home by three, and he was nervous. Gregg seemed fine, and that increased Anthony's anxiety even more. Maybe they should just keep on like they had been doing. They both knew all the players well, they liked all of the staff at Dr. Martin's office, and it was easier each time to get in and out of the hospital, since they had been there a number of times before. Why should they introduce all these new people at a time when things were complicated enough already? It seemed like a thousand more "Why?" questions raced through his mind before the doorbell rang at 3:55 P.M. These hospice people were even going to be early. It was clear they knew nothing about the people they were visiting!

A man and a woman appeared at the door, introducing themselves as Jan Krueger, the hospice nurse, and David Ashford, the social worker, who specialized in care for people with AIDS.

Gregg indicated he had read a brochure about hospice that his physician had given him, and shared quickly that he had forgotten to give this brochure to Anthony to read, so perhaps they could review the basics, even though he thought he understood them. If they started at the beginning, everyone would have the same information—perhaps not the same understanding, but at least the same information.

Jan started with an overview of hospice services. David talked about other people they had cared for, and shared some stories, which were really quite helpful and comforting even if everyone did die.

Anthony had lots of questions about his role. What happened when he had to go to work? How comfortable would the hospice people be coming into their home? Could team members be replaced if it wasn't working? What happened if things changed and Gregg got better? He also had quite a few questions that he was able to ask David alone, while Jan was talking with Gregg.

Anthony understood the "not hastening death" aspect of the hospice philosophy, but had a number of questions about the "not postponing death" part. David explained that hospice would be working with them to assess Gregg's quality of life through each step of the process. Everything would be discussed and considered. Each OI would be looked at individually, and David once again provided an array of examples that gave comfort to Anthony.

Unlike many people, Gregg and Anthony had completed all of their paperwork. Gregg had been particularly compulsive about the paperwork issue. Lots of their friends had ended up in a real mess because nothing was on paper. They both had wills, they had both signed appropriate health care and financial power of attorney, and they would update their living will paperwork on the next visit.

In his own mind Gregg was still working, although the university had switched him from a teaching schedule to a research schedule for the semester, and he hadn't been to the office for any length of time for nearly a month. He was still accessing the research network from home, reading, and writing several papers for publication, but even that was lessening.

David and Anthony helped him to transition to the disability program provided by the school, assuring that his insurance remained intact and that financially they were going to be okay—fortunately.

Gregg thought about cashing in his insurance policy from the university, which was fairly sizable. But after he thought more about it and he and Anthony talked about it, there wasn't anything grand he really wanted to do, and he didn't need the financial resources. And besides, the policy was written to be shared on a percentage basis between Anthony and Gregg's family, so it might be less messy just to leave it for now. He could reconsider down the line if he needed to.

Gregg wasn't in need of a great deal of physical assistance and care at this point, so it was decided that Jan only needed to come once a week for now. Things really felt pretty comfortable. Gregg felt that Anthony was supportive of his decision—*their* decision, really—and he had a degree of comfort with the people involved so far. That was actually a great relief to Gregg. Also, he didn't get the feeling from Anthony that he just wanted this to be over. They both recognized that this was another dose of reality that goes with the disease, even for long-term survivors.

A calm and comfortable routine ensued, with David's weekly visit bringing up some of the gray areas. Gregg was wrestling with when to tell his family that things had changed. He was hoping against hope that this too might pass, but he did not want to miss this important time with them, either. He talked with them on the phone on a regular basis, just as he always had. No need to change that. He just left out the part about being sick. He had been home two years ago during the summer, and he wasn't planning to go home until next summer. They would want to come if they knew. They would get in the car and drive all eight hundred miles right after he called or wrote, and probably never want to leave. What would Anthony do? Their previous visits had all been touring visits, a day or two, sightseeing and then on their way.

But in the back of his mind, Gregg knew that even if they would come immediately, he did want time with them. He clearly had to have the conversation. It was one of those conversations that he had held in his head a thousand times over, but it just didn't gel like he wanted it to, so it didn't ever happen.

All of Gregg's family acknowledged Anthony and made him feel very warmly welcomed, and Anthony's family certainly had responded in the same way toward Gregg. The situation, the arrangement, the realness of the relationship just hadn't been discussed. Gregg's philosophy had been that they probably already knew, after this long of a time, and that if they were really ready to know, and ask, he would tell them. This situation somewhat complicated the issue.

Gregg spent quite a bit of time thinking about the "What ifs" related to the conversation. The only thing David was pushing for, and Gregg realized it after a few weeks, was for Gregg to be sure of what he wanted to do. This was not a sideline event, it was center field, and if he wanted time with his family while he could most enjoy it, the conversation was of utmost importance.

Gregg authored a script in his head, and even keyed a script on the screen of his computer, but never saved it. Maybe Anthony could call—he would have to call anyway if Gregg got worse, was taken to the hospital, or couldn't talk. Or, better yet, maybe David should call, as he had clearly done it before.

No, it was a call he had to make himself. He obviously

knew his family would be distressed, but the only thing they would be really mad about was that he hadn't told them before this time, that he and Anthony had handled this by themselves for all this time. Why? He didn't have an answer for that one yet; it had just been easier. He hadn't ever been really dangerously ill with an OI. Only a couple of times was he close to having Anthony call them, and then he got better, so there wasn't really a reason to worry them. This time, however, it was a little beyond creating worry. It was about time, and this disease wasn't·a cooperating player with any sort of prediction. He also knew he didn't want to take the chance of easing into dementia, of being here and not being here from time to time, an experience he had seen in a number of his friends.

As with any difficult conversation, there were lots of tears, and three or four calls that followed that same day and during the next few days. Gregg persuaded his family not to get in the car and head out that day, but to work with him and with Anthony to support some resemblance of a schedule. Gregg dealt best with the known, and schedules helped him to have some level of control. Anthony also received a number of calls at his office from Gregg's mother. She needed reassurance about Gregg's care. She clearly recognized Anthony's role in the relationship, even without "the talk" that Gregg thought would be needed.

Anthony did his best to meet everyone's needs, to welcome Gregg's family and his work associates. Gregg didn't have any desire for another trip back home. Anthony was a little relieved, although he would have done it gladly. Gregg said that he got out once, and that he didn't want to take the chance of going back and being sick and not being able to get out again. He always added.a little humor to his decisions.

Gregg's mother's visits were more frequent as the weeks went on, and she stayed an additional day each time she came, but Anthony actually got so he looked forward to her being there. This had not been the experience of many of their friends with similar situations, so they were even more appreciative of the strength that all of Gregg's family brought to their home.

Gregg had been spared any terrible battles with Kaposi's sarcoma, thrush, or any of the other common opportunistic infections. He did have ongoing challenges with pneumonia. He had what he felt had been six different types of pneumonia, and rather than try to deal with the details, he referenced his ongoing problem as CF—chest fluid—and that had to be good enough for anyone who asked.

Gregg was always kept comfortable. He took the hospice team seriously when they said he should never be in pain. If he was in pain, he was to tell them about it. For the most part, pain was prevented and never became a real concern. Gregg worried more about Anthony than anything else. He was sure at this point he probably wouldn't tell him how he was really coping, but he seemed to be hanging in there okay.

Anthony was in fact doing okay. He tried to spend all the time he could with Gregg, even though it was difficult to see his partner get weaker and sicker. He valued the time they had. He relied heavily on the hospice team and buddies for support and guidance—exactly what they told him to do. He maintained a routine work schedule as much as possible, although his employer had granted him some additional flexibility in his schedule to care for Gregg. He knew he would need that flexibility in the near future, as things were changing fairly quickly now.

Gregg had gotten so he loved the sofa; he had a grand view of the city from the living room window. He knew a hospital bed would have been easier, probably better for everyone else, but he so hated the thought of how it would be in the living room.

Gregg died peacefully on the living room sofa on a Saturday afternoon, with Anthony close by. Without fanfare, without struggle, and without drama, peacefully and quietly, even unexpectedly to a point. One never knows when death will actually occur. Anthony held Gregg quietly for a while, then called Jan and David, who seemed to handle things from there. Anthony called Gregg's family, and said he would call back later in the day when he could talk about the arrangements Gregg wanted.

This was one area where Gregg did print the brief script he had written and had shared with Anthony, indicating his desire for cremation, and an uplifting memorial service with their friends and colleagues in the city, with a reception at their apartment to follow. He also knew it would be important for his family to have another memorial service in his hometown, and wanted Anthony to be sure his family knew he was fine with that, if they wanted to do so. Gregg requested that half of his ashes be interred in the family cemetery plot, and the other half scattered wherever and whenever Anthony wanted to do so.

This was, ironically, memorial service number one hundred for Anthony. He'd sworn that when he got to a hundred he wouldn't go to another. He'd thought he would be numb by this time, but found it wasn't the case at all. He realized that even though it was in fact uplifting, as he had promised Gregg it would be, he ached with pain. He quickly realized why Gregg had requested the reception at home: it helped Anthony to be in their own home, with friends and family around, to socialize, and remember Gregg's life.

Anthony wasn't sure he could attend the memorial service in Gregg's hometown, or if it might be better that he not. In the notes Gregg had left, he asked him to go if he could, but said everyone would understand if he couldn't. He had only been there one time, and that was over four years ago, and only for a long weekend on the way back from somewhere.

Anthony had talked at length with Gregg's family during these past few months. He had been in touch with them almost daily since Gregg's death to talk through with them the notes that Gregg had left regarding services and arrangements.

Gregg's mother sent the local paper with Gregg's obituary, and indicated they were planning a simple square marker for the cemetery, unless he thought differently. Anthony really wasn't interested in the cemetery marker, but it was nice of her to ask just the same. What really caught his attention was his name in the obituary. It was something he certainly was not expecting. The obituary was well written, with both feeling and facts, listing names of survivors one and all. No titles were necessary. Everyone in that little town knew that Robert and Nancy Johnson were Gregg's parents, so they didn't need to be announced, and that Tamara was Gregg's sister. For those who did know Anthony Carson, he was proud to be included, and for those who didn't know who Anthony Carson was, it didn't matter. He smiled, and picked up the phone to call Gregg's mother, to check in to see how they were doing, and to thank her.

Aspects of Dying with AIDS

As a disease, AIDS (acquired immune deficiency syndrome) generates fear, judgmentalism, and misunderstanding. Most people have little knowledge of AIDS, and that lack of knowledge creates an averse response to persons living with AIDS (PLWA).

At the close of the twentieth century, AIDS is now a disease that is increasingly affecting females, heterosexuals, infants, adolescents, and people spanning all cultural and socioeconomic groups. While there have been significant advances in extending life for persons living with AIDS, the disease still typically ends in death.

The care plan for this disease continues to change. The introduction of protease inhibitors has changed the profile of disease management a great deal. Although these drugs have been successful for the vast majority of patients who can access them, there does exist a group of people, like Gregg, for whom they have been unsuccessful in arresting the progression of the disease.

UNDERSTANDING HIV DISEASE
Cultural Avoidance and Denial

For many reasons, there has been major avoidance and denial surrounding AIDS. These reasons include the fact that HIV seems to have first appeared (or reappeared) far away in Africa, that the original victims of the disease were homosexuals or intravenous drug users—both marginalized members of society—and that the infection typically does not emerge until eight to eleven years following infection. All of these factors led to the sense that the disease was not a concern to most people. The spread of the disease is still surrounded by denial and avoidance.

Families and AIDS

The stigma associated with homosexuality in many areas of the country and in many religious and cultural traditions makes it difficult for many gay men to tell their family of origin that they are homosexual. Gregg had never directly told his parents that he was gay, or that he was HIV-positive. Many persons living with AIDS and their significant others are unsure of the response they might receive from various members of their families of origin.

Gay children are often estranged from their family of origin. In many families, even those who have positive relationships like Gregg's, the news of advanced AIDS is the first news the family has received not only about the disease, but about sexual orientation. Many persons living with AIDS feel that they must keep the fact that they have this disease from their family of origin until the time that they may actually be dying from it. Families of origin may also have misinformation and heightened fear of possible contagion and transmission.

Two Families

Gregg and Anthony each had two families, as most of us do: family of origin, and family of choice. Many adults in our mobile and transient American society move away from their family of origin and live with their family of choice. The relationships between these families intersect in different ways at different times for all of us. A life-threatening illness and death of a family member brings together these two families, sometimes in expansive ways and sometimes in controlling or excluding ways. When the family of choice involves a gay couple, the dynamic between the family of origin and the family of choice can often be challenging from a variety of perspectives.

There may also be tension and rivalry between the family of origin and the family of choice. In some cases, the family of origin can be overtly rejecting and exclude the family of choice. Competition over certain roles or the existence of long-standing grievances add to the complex dynamic and can give rise to major hostilities between the family of origin and the family of choice. Some family members maneuver for status and positions of importance during the last stages of the illness and the dying process. Hospice professionals can help encourage cooperation and collaboration among all family members.

Hospice and Families

Traditionally, hospice care has operated with a broad definition of family that includes those who are in close relationships with the person who is dying—those people who the individual defines as family. In AIDS care, this approach can sometimes be complicated by a struggle over control and decision-making between the two families.

While comfortable, mutual respect is not always the experience when the two families come together, it can help to bridge some of the feelings of pain, competition, and diminishment that are typically present. Ultimately, families do best who focus in on the love and care of the person who is ill, rather than on competition based on individual roles and relationships. Models of competent and collaborative care for persons who die of AIDS exist and need to be encouraged.

In addition to advancing cooperative models of care, hospice encourages the qualities that help families live through the painful loss of a loved one. Families who are able to survive tragedies possess some notable characteristics:

1. Refusing to be bitter
2. Living in the present; coping with the crisis at hand
3. Managing conflicts creatively
4. Allowing one another room to breathe
5. Protecting one another; sheltering from further harm[1]

Gregg's two families consistently showed these characteristics. Not all families can live up to ideal characteristics. The family patterns and degree of openness are what brings out workable approaches even in painful times.

When the person who is ill and dying is gay, he is often a member of a larger community of gay men and women who have supported each other across time. Part of the network of support for persons living with AIDS is a committed group of friends and neighbors who share information, bring food, run errands, provide care, and encourage the ill person and the family members present.

Communication

Facilitating end-of-life communication is one of the important services that hospice offers to families. Almost all families struggle with misunderstandings and deficits as they face the death of a loved one. In spite of his hesitations and concerns, things worked out well when Gregg told his family of origin about his illness. Talking with an objective, experienced per-

son like the hospice social worker, David, saved Gregg some
of the time and energy he was spending on worrying.

Most people find it useful to have some help sorting
through what is important when choices and decisions are
pressing. If Gregg had spoken earlier with the hospice social
worker or nurse, he might have chosen to talk to his family
sooner. The many concerns that Gregg and Anthony juggled
added to their stress. Anthony was actually relieved to have
Gregg's mother and family help with his care. It's a large
undertaking to handle alone.

One of hospice's key actions can be to encourage and
facilitate the involvement of all family members, acknowledging each person's importance to their dying loved one. One of
the successes in Gregg's experience centered around the way
Gregg's family worked *with* Anthony to care for Gregg, each
encouraging and honoring the other's involvement.

Changes and Needs

AIDS changes so many aspects of a person's life, physically,
emotionally, financially, and spiritually. Just like people who
live with cancer, there is also a great deal about persons living
with AIDS that doesn't change: their basic personalities and
characters, concerns about relationships, careers, and families;
and all the other struggles that we engage in on a day-to-day
basis.

Mary Fisher is an eloquent advocate and a "pilgrim on
the road to AIDS." Raised in a socially prominent Michigan
family, she had a successful career that included being Gerald
Ford's first "advance man," a television producer, and an
artist. Her world transformed when she learned her former
husband had AIDS and that she had been infected and was
HIV-positive. Fisher talks about the parts of people's lives
that are not changed by AIDS, like the need for affection and
acceptance, for the delights in the experience of living, and
for continuing and sustaining relationships. Persons living

with AIDS still fear death, but that fear is balanced out, as it is for all people who are dying, by feeling loved and valued.

> *What doesn't change, of course, is our need to be human. To have purpose. To feel the touch of someone's hand. To know that, if we were gone, someone would notice and care. To imagine that we might have made a difference. To believe that someone will remember us.*
>
> —MARY FISHER, 1995[2]

Hospices and AIDS Care

Hospices have traditionally cared for persons dying from cancer, where there is a predictable course of the disease and treatments associated with it. Approximately 60 percent of all care provided by hospice programs is provided to persons with cancer. In 1994, hospices cared for 37 percent of all people who died of cancer-related causes in the United States, and for 31 percent of all who died of AIDS-related causes. In some communities, however, hospice has a care rate of over 90 percent of those who die of cancer and almost 70 percent of those who die of AIDS.[3]

Because AIDS typically is a progressively chronic disease with an unpredictable trajectory, it requires specialized care and services from hospices. The roller-coaster nature of the illness, with acute episodes and recovery, makes the prognosis of six months or less of life difficult to predict. The advent of protease inhibitors has meant that PLWAs who take the medication are able to stay active and healthier longer. When death occurs, it is often as a result of a rapidly occurring opportunistic infection.

Gregg was among the group of people who do not respond to the new protease inhibitors. He lived in a large urban area with access to health care and hospice professionals who were very familiar with the needs of the person living with AIDS, and with AIDS care in general. Had Gregg chosen to stay with his family of origin in the rural area where they lived, the health care professionals and hospice professionals would typically have less skills and information related to end-of-life care for PLWAs. They would typically access current information from other programs that care for larger numbers of persons with AIDS. Currently, the majority of AIDS care takes place in major metropolitan areas. Rural hospices struggle more with having adequate staff training and experience. Families in rural areas caring for a PLWA also have unique needs around the right of confidentiality, desires for secrecy, and possible social isolation. When care is provided in rural areas, resource information is available from the National Hospice Organization and from experienced metropolitan hospice programs.[4]

Barriers to Accessing Hospice Care

There are numerous other barriers to the access of hospice services by persons living with AIDS, including the fact that many of the persons living with AIDS are young people. Referral resources are often reluctant to introduce hospice services as an alternative. One of the ethics that AIDS service organizations promote is "fighting the good fight." Some see hospice as giving up the fight. Also, like people struggling with advancing cancer, many young persons living with AIDS could see utilizing hospice services as giving up hope. Some AIDS service organizations and other community providers may have misperceptions about hospice, believing that it is meant for those who have relinquished hope and discontinued treatment. Or, other providers may choose to maintain their relationship with their AIDS clients rather than lose their connection with them. Finally, a disproportionate percentage of the current population of persons living with AIDS are African-American or Hispanic. Traditionally, these minority groups mistrust medical institutions and have difficulty accessing appropriate services.

From the hospice program perspective, some hospices still have admission requirements for the presence of a primary caregiver. Many persons living with AIDS do not have a caregiver living in the home. Some hospice programs also have concerns about the possibility of financial burdens the hospice might experience in providing care to persons living with AIDS. Hospices that utilize the Medicare or Medicaid benefit for the care of a PLWA are responsible for most medications. The many medications, including those to treat OIs, can place a financial burden on the hospice. Alternative sources of funding, such as grants and donations, must be sought to underwrite costs.

In addition, because the demographics of persons living with AIDS includes intravenous drug users and gay men, there can be emotional and prejudicial responses from a broad spectrum of people—including referral sources and hospice service providers—that could limit access to hospice services.

Hospice Bereavement Programs

Just as prejudice and shame can limit access to hospice services, they can also give birth to significant distress for surviving partners and relatives. Hospice bereavement services and programs can be of particular importance when surviving family members have limited support which they feel they can access. The bereavement services that a hospice offers to an individual or family are based upon a *bereavement assessment* that includes:

- Social, religious, cultural, and gender influences
- The survivors' needs
- Individual history and concurrent experiences of grief and loss
- Risk factors
- Potential for pathological grief reactions[5]

One of the key determinants of outcome following the death of a loved one is the availability of social support. The absence of support, or social isolation, is seen as a major element of risk for the bereaved. People who have lost family members or partners due to AIDS have major additional vulnerabilities.[6, 7] Many people who die from AIDS are young, so their death means the loss of a child, sibling, or contemporary. A young person's death can create individual or family conflicts involving unresolved developmental tasks. In addition to the element of untimely death, people who lose a loved one to AIDS can be depleted by caregiving during the protracted illness. Even with the success of protease inhibitors, a death from an opportunistic infection can happen in a number of days, leaving family members shocked at the suddenness of their loved one's death.

Working with Accumulated Losses

For some members of gay communities, there is an accumulation of all the deaths and losses that they have experienced over recent years. These can actually number a hundred or more, creating a situation not unlike battle-zone conditions, where survivors feel surrounded by death. Multiple losses require different adaptations from the bereaved. The typical assumption that healthy responses to grief involve expression and exploration of the meaning of the loss is not realistic in this context. Looking too closely at a recent loss experience can tap into all the other losses and create a feeling of being flooded or overwhelmed with grief. The grief may actually feel too large to take in at any one point in time.

Situations of multiple loss can be better dealt with indirectly, in small doses, when the person feels able to acknowledge some part of the experience. Otherwise, it is important to keep the grief in the background so that it does not incapacitate the person. The comfort for multiple losses is found when the grieving person can receive support and understanding without major exploration. When considering multiple losses, integration of the losses may not be a realistic goal, since there is literally too much to absorb. Rather, the image of sitting with the losses and looking at them with sidelong glances may be more appropriate.

Art and rituals are two ways that have been found to be particularly helpful and comforting to those who have lost many loved ones. The AIDS quilt is a focal point for many bereaved partners and family members. It offers an opportunity to recognize and memorialize in a personal way the loved one who has died. Also, viewing the quilt in exhibit can help acknowledge the magnitude of the losses and the shared grief that is linked and stitched together, like the panels, accompanying it everywhere it goes.

Challenges

Working with persons with AIDS challenges hospice programs to offer bereavement services that take into account the unique needs of the survivors of persons who have died. The assessment process needs to address their individual concerns, including possible issues around shame, support, and substance abuse. The typical supportive services and groups may not be effective for those bereaved through AIDS. In larger communities where additional services are available, coordinated efforts with AIDS service organizations and other community groups are desirable. Hospices typically offer preventive, educational, and supportive services for the first year of bereavement. That time frame may not be sufficient, just as it often is not for the other bereaved family members that hospices serve. Hospices should focus on their best supportive efforts, given the circumstances and time available, and also refer survivors to other outside resources.

Serving the "Looking-Glass Community"

At the October 1993 annual symposium of the National Hospice Organization, Mary Fisher made three requests of the collected hospice care providers. First, she urged them "to open the doors of hospice not only to the *promise* of care for those with AIDS, but to the *reality.*" Her second request was "Simply that you see those who are my fellow pilgrims on the road to AIDS for what we are: a looking-glass community. We are the people who, when someone dies of AIDS, see ourselves and our future." Mary Fisher's third and final "simple request" was that hospices serve not only those who are now pilgrims on the road to AIDS, "but also our children."[8] Many lives and years have been lost to the disease of AIDS. Many more will be lost. The disease challenges hospices and communities to follow their values and principles by offering the most humane and expert services to these underserved people.

No man is an island, entire of it self; every man is a piece of the continent, a part of the main; if a clod be washed away by the sea, Europe is the less, as well as if a promontory were, as well as if a manor of thy friends or of thine own were; Any man's death diminishes me, because I am involved in mankind.

—JOHN DONNE
"No Man Is an Island"

Chapter Ten

SHATTERED DREAMS
A Community Responds to a
Tragic Accident

· Who would ever expect that a busload of high school students headed for the girls state indoor soccer tournament would crash? It happened on February 26, two hours out of Springfield, on Highway 127. With good weather and clear roads, the bus was ahead of schedule. The plan was to reach Castle Pines before 9 P.M. so the players could get a good night's sleep before the next day's 8 A.M. game. They were excited about the finals, and confident of placing in the top three.

It was a two-lane road, and there wasn't a lot of traffic. The pickup came from out of nowhere. Police estimated that it was going over 70 mph. At first, he crowded close to the back of the bus, pushing it to go faster. There was no place to pull over, and there was a double yellow line. This went on for a minute or two, then the pickup swung into the opposite lane. He hadn't seen the oncoming car. Everything happened so fast after that.

The pickup tried to get back in the lane to avoid the car, but there was no place to go. The car overcorrected to avoid the pickup. The car's driver lost control and crossed the road, crashing into the front side of the bus. Swerving to avoid the car, the pickup bumped into the back side of the bus. At 55 mph, the bus driver did all he could to control the bus, but it went off the road. Traveling over the rough shoulder and the edge of a ravine, the bus rolled on its side and crashed engine-first into the deep ditch.

A sixteen-wheeler was approaching from the opposite direction and saw the bus roll off the road. The noise was so loud, the truck driver felt it shake him. As soon as Bill Shakworth could stop his huge machine, he was on the CB calling for help. Then he jumped down from the truck and ran over to the bus. There was a lot of screaming and crying from inside. The bus had landed against its right side and there was no way to reach the door. He climbed onto the left side of the bus and called in through a broken window. There was so much fear and panic he almost couldn't stand it. Just as he was about to get a couple of the kids to climb out through the window, he heard the sirens. He told them he would stay with them, that help would be here in a minute or two.

The next thing Bill remembers is seeing the stumbling driver of the pickup. He had several cuts on his head and arms, and he smelled strongly of whiskey. He rambled on about not seeing the car, and said to Bill, "I guess I ruined my truck." It was all Bill could do to hold back from hitting him, but he knew that he was drunk, and saw the highway patrol officer walking toward them. In the background, there were already four or five teenagers who the officers had removed from the bus lying on the ground at the side of the road. The patrol officer held back the pickup driver, who was insisting on going over to help the students.

George Stokes, a county sheriff's officer, was the first law enforcement official on the scene. Based on the police report, they had already put out a four-county disaster alert about the accident, and now the full disaster response was in motion. They set up a triage at the accident scene. The local hospital was twenty-one miles away in Brighton and was the primary treatment site. Ambulances, medical professionals, and emergency personnel were called from as far away as Brownsville. Emergency workers had never seen anything like it locally.

There were casualties everywhere, and several of the young people were already dead.

It was just before 8:30 P.M. when the call came in to the Hillside Hospice answering service. They immediately contacted John Anderson, Carol Studerbach, and Gary Neilson at their homes. Two years before, Hillside Hospice had hosted a county initiative to develop a master plan for disaster response. At the hospice's invitation, sixty-two first responders and associated helping professionals came together to plan for a situation such as this. Representing the full range of law enforcement and medical, psychological, spiritual, and other helping professionals in the county, they had all hoped that they would never have to use the disaster-response plan. Now, when they needed it, it was a relief to know that everything was in place. Everyone was clear about their roles, coordination was established, and backup was already called from the surrounding counties.

Gary Neilson had been working with Hillside Hospice for seven years, and before that had volunteered with them for two years. As the Hospice chaplain and coordinator of bereavement services, he had established a broad network of groups and services for the community at large, not just hospice families. A veteran of Vietnam, Gary had a great deal of experience with trauma. If there was one thing that he had learned serving in the army, it was that you get through difficult times together, by helping each other in whatever ways possible. That battalion or, as he would refer to it now, *community* approach to survival offered the best chances and most possibilities for getting through dangerous times.

Gary's role on Springfield's Disaster-Response Team was threefold. He was one of five people notifying the families. Since the accident had occurred ninety-five miles from Springfield, he was also one of the people coordinating transportation for the family members to Brighton General Hospital. Finally, in the months and years that would follow, Gary would coordinate the support groups offered to the grieving families, as well as to the survivors.

The notification team gathered at the Springfield Police Department. After they made the initial round of calls, one team member stayed at the police department and four drove family members to Brighton. Gary drove Marie Cozetto and Anna Rodriguez to Brighton in his car. It was the longest two-hour drive he could ever remember. Anna was a single parent, and her youngest daughter, Louisa, was the star forward on the team. Marie Cozetto had two sons and two daughters, and Patricia, her oldest, was playing on the team for the first time. There were questions and tears, and chunks of deep silence as the three rode on, not knowing what to expect.

Carol Studerbach, a hospice nurse and emergency responder, had grown up in Springfield. Except for five years away at the university for her bachelor's degree in nursing, she had stayed in the area. Her career began in medical surgical nursing, and then she went on to work on the intensive care unit and the emergency department. Almost three years before she had joined Hillside Hospice as a nurse, and this year she'd become the patient-care coordinator. Finally, she felt that she'd found her place in nursing.

When Gary asked Carol if she was interested in the Disaster-Response Team work, she thought it was a good blend of her technical skills and her hospice work. She believed that hospice needed to broaden its services to the community, and this was a natural opportunity. Her role was to be involved with triage at the hospital and, later, to offer on-site support for the nursing team. After the call came in, Carol went to the Springfield Community Hospital and waited at the emergency department for word about the transfer of patients. Since they were two hours away, it wasn't clear if another team would be transported to Brighton. A team of three doctors and three nurses had been flown by helicopter an hour before, and now they were waiting for further word. Carol was on the second team scheduled to depart.

John Anderson, the third hospice responder, was a licensed clinical psychologist in private practice who worked as a consultant to the Hillside Hospice team. He had been involved with Hillside Hospice since it originated eighteen years earlier. In his role as consultant, he sat in on the weekly interdisciplinary team meetings and ran the biweekly staff-support meetings. He also occasionally met individually with staff members who were having difficulties related to their hospice work.

When the police and sheriff's departments started their victim-advocate programs, John was very involved in the planning, as well as in the training of the advocates. He had also conducted some debriefing sessions and support meetings for the police and sheriff's departments. Because his work had focused on post-traumatic stress and on the ways helping professionals cope with stress, he was interested in being a part of the disaster planning efforts. When Gary had invited John, he became committed to the group. John's role was to be available to officers and medical personnel who were at the scene responding to the accident and caring for the victims of the crash. He would hold debriefing sessions at the Brighton site, and afterward in Springfield.

The tragedy was worse than anyone could have expected. Five teenage girls were dead at the scene of the accident, seven other girls were in critical condition with major injuries, and six students had sustained moderate or slight injuries. Both the driver of the bus and the driver of the car were severely injured. Those with moderate injuries were moved by ambulance back to Springfield within two hours. Extra staff were brought in to work with the critically injured, and they would not be moved until they stabilized.

Hospital staff helped the coroner set up extra rooms so that the families of the girls who'd died could see them and spend time with their bodies. Gary was part of the group of chaplains and mental health professionals who'd comforted the families of the girls who died at the scene. They met with the families at Brighton General, offering support to them during those first terrible hours.

There were many behind-the-scenes arrangements going

on. After a call from the hospital about the number of fatalities involved and the distance from their hometown, funeral directors from both Brighton and Springfield worked out special arrangements for the transportation of the bodies of the girls who had died. There were countless ways that the surrounding communities worked together to make the aftermath of the tragedy as uncomplicated as possible for the families.

The crisis responses to the bus crash were like the connected spokes on a wheel. The people in need were at the center of the wheel, with support people from various agencies all focusing on that center, offering services to the many people involved. According to the disaster plan, all the efforts were coordinated and all the major needs were addressed with every responder fulfilling their designated role—some aiding those on the scene and in the hospitals, some notifying and supporting the families, some planning services geared toward the long-term grief of the families, and, finally, some setting up supportive efforts aimed at the accident's impact on the helping professionals.

Two days after the crash, Gary called a meeting to evaluate the effectiveness of the plan, and each component of the operation. Forty of the responders involved broke into small groups and discussed the elements of their participation that worked as planned, and those that could be improved in the future. At that meeting, John had also arranged for a psychiatrist from a neighboring town to do an additional debriefing with them. John knew that because of his close involvement in the crash response, an outside resource was needed for subsequent debriefings. The meeting began with the first officers on the scene and the investigating officers describing in detail their best reconstruction of the crash.

One of the most difficult aspects of the crash was that the loss of life and injury involved teenage girls aged fourteen to seventeen. Because Springfield is a town of just over 60,000 people, it seemed almost everyone knew someone affected by the crash. Some of the people involved in the crisis response found they were working with neighbors, members of their church community, people they identified with a great deal. That made the impact greater, and the toll on the responders was larger than they anticipated. There was a lot of open discussion and emotion when the crash was discussed. The law enforcement officers talked forcefully about their anger at the drunken driver, and their frustrations with the legal system. Many of those who spoke talked about feelings of helplessness and powerlessness in the situation.

One of Hillside Hospice's ongoing services was a bereaved parents group where the parents of the students would be invited by another bereaved parent to participate. In addition, Hillside Hospice supplied staff and volunteers to the local high schools to participate with school counselors in student assemblies held after the crash. Volunteers were also cofacilitators of a student loss group that was scheduled for eight weeks each semester. Finally, for several months following the bus crash, Hillside Hospice staff organized and participated in debriefing meetings for the crises responders.

Gary, Carol, and John met twice after the crash to discuss their own involvements, and to look at the role that Hillside Hospice had played in the overall community response. The following month they were to present a report and recommendations for future activities to the hospice board. They all agreed that the feedback about hospice's efforts had been overwhelmingly positive. The responders saw hospice as the originator of the coordinated disaster-response plan, as an important participant in the on-the-scene services, and also as the key provider of supportive bereavement services to the families.

When Gary, Carol, and John met together, they each spoke of the differences and similarities between trauma responses and their hospice care experiences. While families caring for their loved ones are often worn down by the process and progression of the illness, there are relatively few surprises. Trauma not only involves physical devastation, it usually means an unexpected, extraordinary event, even a disaster, has occurred. Gary, Carol, and Bob all felt that their work in hospice had helped them handle this trauma-response experience. They felt it was good to work with a team approach, just as hospice care involves teamwork.

The last thing that Gary, Carol, and Bob each spoke about were the stories about the injured young people, the distraught parents, and the responders who struggled with the horror of the scene.

"It's the people who died, and the family members who love them. I still see the faces and relive some of the things people said. I suppose that is all that really matters in the work that we do, whether it's a cancer death or a violent, sudden death," Carol reflected.

"I know," Gary added. "I keep thinking about Ms. Cozetto, who I drove to Brighton. She and Mrs. Rodriguez talked in the car on the way to Brighton about their daughters, Patricia and Louisa. Patricia was dead and Louisa has severe injuries. I went to Patricia's funeral. It was heart-wrenching to see her parents and brothers and sisters. It's an image I won't forget. The young people who were the pallbearers cried all the way into the church and out, too. I plan to call Ms. Cozetto next week. I still think what a random world it is where one daughter dies and the other lives—what a fine line there is between living and dying. Again, I'm reminded that life is so unpredictable and like a thin thread that is easily broken."

> *As far as we can discern, the sole purpose of human existence is to kindle a light in the darkness of mere being.*
>
> *—CARL JUNG*

Hospice Bereavement Services

At their outset, hospice programs grew from unmet needs related to the dying process. Perhaps the most unique element of hospice services lies in the inclusion of the family as the focus of care and services. Related to this principle of a family-centered focus, bereavement follow-up is the component of hospice services that is typically not found in other approaches to end-of-life care.

Hospices offer a unique model of bereavement care and services to families for a period of at least one year following the death of their loved one. Within hospices, bereavement services have been the least developed and most widely varied in their quality of all hospice services. By their very nature in addressing an individual, time-intensive process, bereavement services have been difficult to define. Adding to the absence of paradigms for the definition and delivery of bereavement services, there are serious financial considerations. In the compromises surrounding the passage of the 1982 legislation that authorized Medicare reimbursement for hospice services, Congress specifically excluded payment for any of the costs associated with bereavement services. Hospices must find outside sources of funding for these services—typically grants and donations. This may, in part, explain the wide variation in the quality and scope of hospice bereavement services.

Hospices are required by regulations to perform a bereavement assessment, typically completed by the nurse, social worker, or chaplain involved in care of a particular family. The purpose of the assessment is to determine those individuals who are at significant health or mental health risk during the time of bereavement. In essence, hospice bereavement services are preventive services seeking to offer education, support, and referrals to families, based upon their individual needs (see bereavement services goals, pp. 107–108).

In conjunction with the assessment, hospices typically offer bereaved family members information about the grief process and invite them to participate in a variety of educational and support group offerings. The most typical bereavement services offered by hospice programs include:

- Written information about the grief process
- Periodic bereavement newsletters
- Invitations to educational meetings
- Invitations to bereavement classes/courses
- Invitations to bereavement support groups
- Periodic visits by a bereavement volunteer
- Phone calls from a hospice staff member or volunteer
- Retreats or camps for children, adolescents, and/or families
- Lending library of books, films, and pamphlets about grief
- Referral to a mental health professional if indicated or desired
- Volunteer opportunities (typically after one year)

Additionally, a number of hospice programs offer speakers to clubs, groups, and schools on grief-related topics. This type of community educational involvement is seen as part of the commitment to the community as well as wise public relations by some hospices. Others, like Hillside Hospice, identify a broad range of community education and bereavement services as part of their mission and chosen services to their community.

Community Bereavement Services

Hospices in North America have developed unique additional services, primarily in the area of bereavement care, that have addressed specific needs in their communities. These services are often offered in collaboration or coordination with other community service providers. Representing the typical philosophical commitment that hospices have to their local community, these services are added-on services that staff must find time and resources to offer. In times of rapid growth of hospice services, or of financial limitations, there can be a tendency to avoid involvement in additional community services.

There are a minority of hospice programs that focus only on terminal care and support of the bereaved families they have served. Many other hospice programs believe that community bereavement services fall within the scope of their mission and add to their visibility, strength, and viability. Others see additional services to non-hospice bereaved persons as outside the realm of their mandate and resources.

In June 1995, a meeting of the International Work Group on Death, Dying, and Bereavement, a select group of professionals concerned with standard setting in the field, was held in Oxford, England. Cicely Saunders, the physician founder of the modern hospice movement, addressed the gathering. She told an anecdote about a group of law enforcement officials who'd recently visited the hospice facility and program that she founded, St. Christopher's Hospice. They attended a special training session on "Breaking Bad News." That effort parallels the involvement of hospices in the United States in sudden-death responses and services. Activities such as this are a natural extension of a hospice's area of expertise.

In many communities, the hospice staff are seen as expert resources on death and grief. The vast majority of hospice programs (87 percent) report that they work with teachers and schools on the issue of student deaths.[1] Most hospices make their support groups, educational mailings, phone contacts, and other bereavement services available to family members in their community who have experienced the sudden death of a loved one. However, responding directly to sudden, traumatic deaths and community disasters is not the typical concern of a hospice program. A 1995 survey showed that only 28 percent of hospice programs returning the questionnaire had a process for responding to traumatic deaths in their communities.[2] Hillside Hospice's trauma response program is a more broad-based and far-reaching community effort than that of most hospice programs in the United States.

Throughout the country and the world, there is increasing interest in disaster services and effective interventions in times of trauma. Sometimes, there may be too many well-intentioned people involved, people who do not have a full understanding of the unique effects of trauma upon human beings. Individual hospice programs are discovering ways they can contribute to compassionate care and understanding of the grief of families experiencing sudden death of a loved one.

Hospices and Sudden, Traumatic Death

While there may be debate over hospice's role in community disasters, there is general agreement upon the need for hospice's response in two types of situations that hospices encounter involving traumatic deaths. The first involves the sudden, unanticipated, or unusually shocking circumstances in the death of a hospice patient. The second involves the death of a hospice staff member or volunteer, either as a hospice patient or under sudden circumstances that would call for offering some specialized bereavement services.

Sudden Death of a Hospice Patient

There is an assumption that patients in a hospice program will die an expected, somewhat predictable death. In fact, there are some unusual situations where the hospice death is in fact sudden or traumatic.

Mr. Haywood had metastatic, invasive neck cancer. He was stable, and expected to live at least several more weeks. Late one afternoon, he started to hemorrhage from his neck wound. The tumor had eroded the carotid artery, and he bled into unconsciousness and died shortly after the hospice nurse arrived. Mrs. Haywood was shocked and distraught over the sight of so much blood. While she had been told that the tumor was encroaching, she believed that her husband would die quietly in a few weeks. She was traumatized by the unexpected and difficult circumstances of his death.

Hospices have a responsibility to offer knowledgeable bereavement support to family members like Mrs. Haywood. It is important for hospice professionals to understand the impact of trauma upon the grief process, and the ways in which trauma is different from the experiences of most of the family members that they serve. Trauma blankets us with a layer of concern and fear that must be dealt with before the grief can be addressed. Earlier, more specific, and more intensive support is usually indicated when traumatic circumstances of death have occurred.

Caring for One of Your Own

Another context for looking at hospices' involvement in traumatic deaths centers around the growing numbers of hospice staff members and volunteers who have themselves become or will become hospice patients. This concern also extends to the immediate family members of hospice staff and volunteers

Hospices and Traumatic Deaths

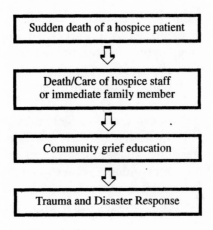

who become recipients of services. These experiences can be considered traumatic because they lie outside the typical experiences and the assumptive worlds of hospice staff and volunteers. The traumatic aspects of these events center around the changed nature of the boundaries, levels of investment and involvement, and the personal impact or toll that these situations exact from hospice workers.

Hospices candidly admit that providing care to one of their own or to the immediate loved one of a staff member or volunteer is one of the more difficult situations that they encounter. It necessitates different patterns of staffing, more complicated staff responses, and additional support and supervision for the hospice-care providers. Dynamics of denial, avoidance, and interpersonal conflicts are all seen when hospices care for their own. Typical assumptions of immunity and attempts to compartmentalize no longer work for hospice-care providers. Outside resources are often indicated to help hospice staffs and volunteers cope with this striking change in circumstances.

Finally, hospice staff members, volunteers, or their immediate family members may also die sudden, violent deaths. The heart attack of a medical director, the stroke that kills a hospice nurse, the fatal automobile accident that kills the daughter of a hospice administrator, or the accidental drug overdose that claims the life of the son of the staff social worker are all examples of sudden, tragic deaths that hospice staffs encounter. Collin Murray Parkes, an English psychiatrist who has conducted important research and written extensively about the grief process, said, "We are the bereaved." In different circumstances and ways, grief will touch all of us.

Hospice workers can come to feel an exaggerated sense of their vulnerability, or that they are surrounded by death. One of the professional adaptations related to hospice work involves the ability to maintain a professional distance and yet be able to offer meaningful, compassionate support. That delicate dance is extremely difficult when a hospice cares for one of its own, or is responding to the death of an immediate family member of a staff person or volunteer. The sudden death of a hospice professional or volunteer or one of their immediate family members precipitates a trauma response in the hospice program and calls for a supportive intervention by an outside resource.

Hospices and Community Grief Education

The third area of hospice involvement in community traumas centers around educating community crisis responders about the grief process. Hospices typically bring together a staff of skilled and experienced professionals who are knowledgeable about the dying and grieving process. Hospice professionals have a great deal of information and understanding about loss and grief to offer other helping professionals who work with sudden deaths. The example Dr. Saunders gave of training law enforcement officers is an apt one. When there is collaboration between helping professionals in a community, both the recipients of services and the professionals benefit. Hospice professionals and volunteers would also profit from knowledge about the trauma response that emergency responder professionals have to offer.

Most hospice programs respond to requests for educational presentations, but unlike Hillside Hospice, they do not initiate or offer them to the community. Increased professional collaboration between hospice professionals and others who work with death and grief-related situations would serve to improve the quality of care and services available to families in times of great personal vulnerability and need.

Trauma and Disaster Response

The fourth and final area of hospice involvement in traumatic deaths centers around participation by members of the hospice team in the actual response to the disaster or deaths. This may be by tangible delivery of crisis support to victims at the scene, or it may mean offering debriefing sessions for those who were involved in the crisis response. Either way, a significant commitment to involvement and ongoing participation in the community response team is made. Only a few hospice programs have initiated this kind of activity. Disasters such as the hurricanes in North and South Carolina, Florida, and Hawaii; flooding in North Dakota, Kansas City, and California; and the bombing of the federal building in Oklahoma City have brought about local hospice involvement because of the loss of lives, even though there was no previous commitment to community trauma support.

Under the umbrella of community trauma support lies not only education of responders, but also group offerings for family survivors of the tragedies. It is most common for hospices to open their bereavement support groups and meetings to any interested members of the community. Special groups for survivors of suicide, bereaved parents, or homicide survivors are also offered by a number of hospice programs across the country. These groups are typically support groups, facilitated either by professionals or trained volunteers.

In an ever-changing health care environment of increasing competition and decision-making about allocation of resources, hospices will be challenged to maintain their commitment to a broad range of community services. It seems only logical that the more hospice programs are integrated into the framework of community services surrounding death and grief, the more successfully the community's needs will be addressed.

To do anything in the world worth doing, we must not stand back shivering and thinking of the cold and danger, but jump in, and scramble through as well as we can.

—SYDNEY SMITH

Chapter Eleven

"I'M A HOSPICE NURSE"
The Costs and Rewards of
Working with Hospice

FOR THE PAST eight years I've worked for Mason County
Hospice. Before that, I worked part-time on a medical/surgical unit
at the local hospital. When I heard that hospice was looking for a
nurse, I told my husband, Tom, that I was going to apply. As usual,
he asked me what it would mean for our family. At the time, our
two children were in high school, and I thought that the daytime
hours would be desirable. When I was on-call in the evenings, my
husband would be at home with the children.

Mostly, I wanted to do home-care nursing, and I felt drawn to
hospice. I've been interested in hospice for a number of reasons.
My dad died of prostate cancer six years ago, and I'd wished that
my mom and I had known about their services. He was in the hospital for his last two weeks, and he often said how much he wanted
to be at home. My mom and I did a pretty good job of taking care
of him before that, but then we just couldn't get his pain and diarrhea under control. I wished hospice could have been available to
us. It seems like a much better way. It would have been a big help
for my mom and dad, and for me, too.

When I interviewed for the hospice position, one of the questions they asked me was, "Why are you interested in hospice nursing?" They seemed satisfied with my reasons and my qualifications. I
know now that they asked that question because it wouldn't be
appropriate to have someone working for hospice who was on a mis-

sion, or who wanted to right past wrongs, or who could only work as a lone ranger. They hired me and I became a part-time hospice nurse.

There is no specific formula for hospice services. We want to address the broad range of needs, and it's similar to offering a family a menu and letting them choose the services that best suit them. Initially, the team typically consists of a nurse, a certified nursing assistant, and a social worker, and we work with the family physician, who is a key influence upon the care. The person who is ill and the family usually have a trusting relationship with their physician. It is important for them not to feel abandoned by the family physician just because a hospice referral was made. The family physician works with our hospice medical director and the nurse on the plan of care, including the medication orders.

Every time I walk up to a home, I am aware that all I really have with me is my nursing bag—and I know that the person who is dying and the family members will need more than I have in that bag. There are so many unknowns in working with a new family, and that can be intimidating. I don't know what to expect, what unique kinds of people they will be. I'm sure the family has similar worries. "Who are these hospice people? Will it be okay to have them visit us in our home? Will they really be able to help us?"

As a hospice nurse, I have learned to be flexible and adapt to the style and needs of the family. One of the bywords that was repeated so often at the hospice team training that I attended was "to meet people where they are." The family makes their choices, and we offer guidance and input.

When I first began with hospice, I did the initial assessment visit along with the social worker or the volunteer coordinator. Now, the hospice patient-care coordinator and the social worker go out to introduce hospice, explain the services and types of payment, and take care of all the paperwork. I'm relieved not to have to do that part, though I miss making the initial contact. I usually go out the next day so that we can move quickly. Time is often short. The average length of our hospice's involvement with a family is thirty-eight days. There's a lot to be done, especially at the outset, so that the family will develop confidence and honestly tell me about their concerns. By the time hospice is called, the family has been through a great deal already, and their resources are often worn pretty thin. I still wish we could get the referrals earlier in the process. That way we could give more substantial help to families sooner.

In working with a family, the first priority is to find out what symptoms are troubling the person who is ill. Hospice care involves vigilant attention to the relief of symptoms. One of the first families I worked with, the Martinez family, taught me a lot about pain- and symptom-management. Mr. Martinez was a very religious man in his early seventies who was in the final stages of bladder cancer that had metastasized to his bones and liver. For some reasons, attached to his religious beliefs and his previous life experiences, he was reluctant to tell us much about his pain or take his medications regularly. After a difficult few days, I sat down with Mr. and Mrs. Martinez to revisit our goals and the plan of care. Mr. Martinez told me that he expected to have pain, that it was part of the cancer. Most of all, he did not want to be sedated or not able to think clearly. We talked for quite a while and we finally worked out a compromise where he agreed to take a lower dose of the pain medication regularly. I also showed him some deep relaxation techniques. After that, the massage therapist visited him twice a week and worked on the muscles in his back to ease some of his pain. Mr. Martinez still had some pain, but much less than before. He seemed to have an idea of what his dying would be like, and even though hospice offered him other possibilities, he chose to do things as he saw best. It's always important to let the person who is ill be the one driving the car in the hospice relationship. My role then becomes the navigator, map reader, or the mechanic. The person who is dying, along with the family, are in control as much as their circumstances allow.

I have also learned so many creative ways to use common sense and home-type remedies, in addition to our best pharmacological agents. That's one of the challenges that I enjoy most: problem-solving ways to make the person comfortable with as little invasion and intrusion as possible. Just the smallest suggestion can save families a great deal of work or worry.

One of the most common worries family members have is when the person no longer has much of an appetite. I let them know that the body has a good reserve and naturally slows down. Fixing the person's favorite foods, milk shakes, or even desserts makes family members feel better. We all associate food with life, so less eating is a frightening sign to the family. People can last for a while without food, and even without fluids. Again, I reassure them that there is no cause for concern, that it is a natural part of the way the body reacts. I suggest that they offer the ill person small amounts of water or a favorite juice throughout the day. I have noticed how much families trust and rely on my experiences. My calm approach gives them more room to be less worried.

I discovered that with each visit I make, I need to keep checking in, asking the person who is ill and the family members about different concerns. Just because they don't tell me doesn't mean that things haven't changed, or that certain worries aren't troubling them. Sometimes things even change between my visits, and then I often hear about them from the nursing assistant or other team members who are involved with the family.

One of the things that I find most unique about hospice nursing is working as part of the interdisciplinary team. I'd never had that much interaction with volunteers or other health care professionals. Now I see it as a real plus. It's helpful to have input and involvement from so many different perspectives. Most of all, I appreciate the support and backup that is what hospice is really all about. Not that it's easy to work as part of a team—sometimes I know it would be quicker if I just went ahead and did things myself. It can be a headache to make so many phone calls, keeping the people involved up-to-date on things. But that's my responsibility and I take it seriously.

I think of caring for a person who is dying and the family members as a puzzle, and all of us who are involved in caring for a hospice family have a different perspective, a different piece of the puzzle. When we put them all together, not only do we get the full picture, but we can also address the larger range of needs that the person who is dying and the family have: physical, emotional, social, and spiritual. And, identifying a need doesn't mean that we have to do it all. I remember working with a woman in her sixties who spoke of her deep spiritual concerns to the nursing assistant, yet refused a visit from the hospice chaplain. She was searching and struggling with questions, but she was not interested in anyone representing an organized religion. The irony is that she spoke about her spiritual questions with the nursing assistant, Maria, who is a Mexican-American and Catholic. The woman knew that, but there was something special in their relationship that made her feel comfortable talking about her searching to Maria. Maria is not one to sell her beliefs. She is a quiet woman who listens a great deal and makes you feel more peaceful just by being around her. Often the ill person chooses who they will tell, and who they want support from in addressing specific concerns.

Each family I work with is unique, and different team members are involved in the care. We have several nursing assistants, two social workers, a part-time chaplain, and several volunteer chaplains. Several times I've asked the dietitian to help me with some complicated digestive problems people encountered. A local pharmacist works with us, and I have consulted with him about a few situations when we couldn't get the pain under control, or where a combination of medications was causing difficulty. There are also occupational and physical therapists we can call upon if their services are needed. A music therapy student established a program for us, and now we have volunteers who offer that service to our families. We have several licensed therapeutic massage therapists who work both with the person who is ill and with the family members. The families I've worked with have genuinely appreciated the comfort and stress-relief of massage therapy.

One of our social workers coordinates the bereavement program, and works with twenty-five volunteers who make home visits and phone calls, host grief educational evenings, and facilitate groups. Last year our hospice worked with three other hospices in the area to offer a bereavement camp for children and adolescents. Another is planned for this summer.

We are fortunate in our community to have many skilled people who serve on our interdisciplinary team, either as paid staff or as volunteers. One of the things that fascinates me is how people see things in such different ways, born out of their experiences as well as the discipline perspective that they represent. There is a lot that we learn from each other, and all the different pieces of the caring puzzle we represent can complement each other, enhancing the care. I have grown to respect the unique contribution that each team member makes, and I appreciate the understanding that they have for the difficulties of my role. Sometimes our roles with a family cross or overlap. Then it's important to communicate and to discuss things clearly at our weekly team meeting. There will always be times when we step on each other's toes. I suppose that's inevitable in home care, especially when we each see the family at different points in time.

Weekly team meetings are our best safeguard for coordinating the care. If I were honest, there are times when a two-hour team meeting seems like too much. There have also been many times when I couldn't wait to get to the meeting to talk about a problem that I was having with the care, or to tell an unusual story about a recent death. Our team focuses on problem-solving at the meetings, and developing or adding to the plan of care. The team meeting is a place where I can gain insight, ideas, and perspectives that may be hard for me to find by myself.

Volunteers are the most unique members of the hospice team. Usually a volunteer will work with only one family at a time, offering friendly visits, running errands, reading to or watching a movie with the ill person, or staying with the ill person while family members get a break. One volunteer that I've worked with several times over the last three years, Jack, is a widower in his early seventies. I remember when he would take the young teenagers in one family on outings to the library for their school projects. He always stopped with them at the music section so that they could select a tape or CD to check out and listen to at home. And he brought cookies for the teens on every visit. That gave him a chance to sit down and talk with them for a bit. The 13-year-old girl once asked Jack if they could adopt each other: "I could use a grandfather like you close by right now."

Three years ago, when my children were both in college, I began to work full-time as a hospice nurse. That means that I typically have eight to eleven families I'm caring for at a given time. Because there are five full-time and two part-time nurses with our hospice, I'm on-call four or five nights a month. Getting up in the middle of the night is not easy, but the families usually don't call unless there is an urgent need.

In my experience, many people die during the evening and the night. My presence can make a big difference to the family around the time of death. Usually we've talked about what the family can expect as their loved one's death nears. When I think that the death may happen within the next two weeks, there is a small pamphlet that I discuss with the family. It describes the changes family members can typically see in their loved one. I leave it with them so that they can look at it when they're able. It helps for people to feel prepared. And, I reassure them that a nurse will be there quickly if they have any concerns.

The vast majority of hospice deaths are quiet, where the person gradually slips away. One of the things that sometimes troubles the family members is the noisy, Cheyne-Stokes breathing that can happen for the last few hours. It sounds labored, but it's usually because the person has taken in less fluids and is not swallowing, so the mucous builds in their throat and rattles.

Being with the family at the time of death is one of the most important services that hospice offers. It is a difficult and almost sacred time. There is a feeling that something very human, and yet also mysterious, has happened. I stay with the family while they say good-bye to their loved one. There are usually soft tears that family members cry. It's not a shock. It's just very sad and hard to see someone you love go.

When they are ready, I call the mortuary. In most cases, the family has previously been in contact with the funeral director of their choice, so the process goes smoothly. Hospice tries to encourage families to make arrangements, if they are ready or able to, in advance of the death. It makes that final time less stressful if those decisions have already been made. Some families can't, so then we help them out as much as possible in considering their choices regarding the arrangements. We are very fortunate to have such helpful funeral directors in our area. In fact, two of them have been active as hospice board members.

The last thing I do before I leave the home is dispose of all the narcotic medications. If there are any small pieces of equipment, frequently I will take them with me when I leave. Then I usually go home and do my final charting on the family. Even if it's during the night, I sit at the kitchen table and finish the paperwork. I found that it wasn't easy to try to fall back to sleep after I got home from a death call. The charting helps me make a transition. Then, I leave voice mail messages for the other members of the team who have worked with the family.

Our hospice encourages the nurse and others involved in the care of a family to attend the funeral. This gives the family the message that they mattered to us as people, and that we acknowledge their loss and their sorrow. Rituals are so important. In my eight years with hospice, I have attended more funerals than I could count. One year I did keep track, and it was forty-three. Hospice nurses see more death in one year than most people see in a lifetime.

Following the death, I visit the family one last time. Usually I pick up any remaining supplies or small equipment. It's a time of closure, of saying good-bye to the family. I try to be sure to tell the person who did most of the caregiving, and any other family members, the things that I noticed about the care they gave their loved one. Even in families where there were difficult or abrasive relationships, I can usually recount a few ways that the person can be credited and complimented. One widow I worked with was angry most of the time. She was almost rough in the way she responded to her dying husband. When I made the visit after he died, I told her that I remembered how many nights she had gotten only a few hours of sleep, and I mentioned how special it was to her husband that she made him his favorite tapioca almost every day, no matter how tired she was. We all need to know that someone thought we did a good job. As the nurse, I'm in a particularly good position to say that to the family members.

The last part of my final visit is to explain to the family about hospice's bereavement services, and to tell them to expect a call from a bereavement volunteer in the next month or six weeks. While I'm not a salesperson, I do let the family know that many people I've worked with have appreciated the hospice bereavement services. Even if they never attended any of the group offerings, they valued some of the written materials about grief, and were glad to receive the phone calls and the monthly bereavement newsletter.

When I go back to the office, I complete the paperwork for the summary, and the assessment, and referral to the bereavement program. Within the next forty-eight to seventy-two hours I will be assigned to a new family. And the story starts again.

There is a standing repartee among people who work in hospice about other people's reactions to what seems to them to be an unusual job or volunteer activity. A classic response is "Oh, I don't know how you can do it. That must be terribly difficult work." Often that ends the conversation, and the person walks away. Another reaction is for the person to proceed to tell you stories about the deaths they have experienced. Finally, a few people react with "Oh, I could never do that. I'm too sensitive to be able to handle it." The implication, of course, is that, since you are able to handle hospice work, you must not be sensitive. Each of these is a variation on the theme of the comments that are often made to people who are grieving. The first response involves a basic acknowledgment, followed by avoidance. In the second reaction, the person is inviting understanding or compassion for his or her own experiences. Finally, there is an attempt to differentiate from you, implying that you are doing something that the person would never see him- or herself doing.

There is a kind of mystique or halo effect that I have seen when people relate to me as a hospice nurse. I think it's because there is so much fear about death. I know that I've changed how I feel about and see life and death.[1] Dying is hard, and yet, it's an important part of life. Dying teaches us a lot about life. I remember a retired metal worker, George, telling me, "You can learn a lot about your own life when you're taking care of people who are dying." I've also been inspired and touched by the strength of the families who have invited me into their homes. It is an enormously challenging and demanding job to care for a loved one who is dying. It's easy to observe all the different ways that people deal with the imminent death of someone they love.

Every person and every family is different. Some of the sharpest points of grief are losing the uniqueness of the person that you loved and losing the completeness of your family. We are all irreplaceable to the people who love us. I've seen what it means to feel anguish in the eyes of a mother whose child dies and in the tears of a husband at the death of his wife of sixty-two years. The emptiness of their world seems almost unbearably cruel.

Death is a large reality, one that is almost impossible to understand or absorb. That's why so many people who are faced with death begin a spiritual search. This is not necessarily a religious journey. It is more of an exploration of the questions "Did my life matter?" "Have I done the things that are important to me?" and "What do I believe will happen when I die?" There is a need for each of us to make peace with our own lives. When all the distractions of work and daily routines are taken away, we focus down to the essential core of our lives.

Spirituality is more important to me now. I have to take the time to reflect on my work and experiences so that I don't lose their potential to remind me of the commitments that I've made in my own life.

Early on, the question "Why?" haunted me a lot. Now I try to feel comfortable not having answers. It's hard to see so many good and kind people struggling with such painful life situations. I know it is not a fair world. It's a random one. I wonder how I will die when the time comes.

I take less for granted now, and I try not to postpone things.

It's important to me to make my stand and work toward the goals that I think matter. There's been a refocusing of my life, and things are clearer now. One widow I worked with talked about the time of her husband's dying as being a "cutting-of-the-cloth time." Some things were no longer important and were cut off. What was left during this difficult time was the part to be cherished.

Hospice has taught me about my own fallibility, about the random nature of illness, and I'm constantly faced with my own limits, with the things that I can do, and all that I cannot. Most of all, there are times when there is little to be done except to keep the person who is dying comfortable and encourage the family to continue to surround the person with caring and love. That may not seem like enough to me sometimes, though I know that it can seem like a great contribution to the family involved.

Hospice work has also taught me a lot about myself and the things that are important to me. On the whole, I'm less materialistic. Things don't matter as much—unless I am using shopping therapy as a way of coping. Being around the kind of physical or emotional suffering that illness and death create makes me grateful for my own health. It's one of the most important gifts we can have in life.

If there is one area that hospice work has affected me most, it's at the relationship level. During my work with hospice, I've met some remarkably good and fascinating people, people I would never have had a chance to know otherwise. There are some people and some families that I will never forget. Not all families are that way to me. I suppose it's only human to relate more to some people than to others. When I am involved with a special person or family, I notice that I give a bit more of myself.

One of the first families that I worked with was an Italian couple in their late sixties. Mary was dying of metastatic uterine cancer, and her husband of forty-three years, Al, was her caregiver. I still remember the tenderness between them. He cared for her physically, cleaned the house, did innumerable loads of laundry, and cooked the meals. She remained cheerful and grateful for all his efforts. Their main focus was to spend as much loving time together as possible. I still can see them sitting in their living room, smiling, with their dog, Rocky, between them. There was such warmth in that home that it was always a treat to visit them, even when she was near the end. Afterward, Al became a hospice volunteer and loved to do errands for families. He was also a host at the monthly bereavement educational evenings. There was a sadness about Al, but he kept on being involved with people. He would say at the bereavement meetings that he missed Mary, and felt lucky to have shared so many years with such a loving woman.

The families who I work with are in a time of their lives where they are open to a supportive stranger. All the layers of fluff that we ordinarily use to buffer us from others are stripped away. Families invite me into the intimacy of their home, and into critical, unforgettable moments of their lives. The unguarded closeness that is part of the process of hospice work made me expect or wish for it in my other relationships. Now I know that we can't live at that level of intensity for long periods of time. It's more possible at the crucial moments of life that are involved in hospice work. We are also safe strangers, who will come and go—we're people where there is no history or emotional obligation attached. That frees the person who is ill and the family to be how they want to be, and allows hospice caregivers to enter into very real human dramas.

Hospice work has affected my relationships. I know how important my family is to me. I have to remind myself not to give all my caring to the families that I am working with. It is just as important for me to love and support my family and friends too. My son tells me that I say "I love you" more since I've worked with hospice. I suppose that we can never hear it often enough.

Working with the hospice team has been a learning experience, but not always an easy one. There are times that I've gotten tired of talking to all the people who are involved with a particular family. Still, I do know that I can't do it all, and the team is not just a great resource, it's also an important source of backup and personal support for me. Our hospice also offers support groups and retreats for us to take the time to look at the costs of this work.

There are occasional conflicts within our hospice team, and times when I feel that the administrators don't make decisions that put the caregiving of families first. Our hospice is like the real world, full of problems and possibilities. When we behave as a team, in concert with the values that hospice represents, then we are at our best. I have found that the basic values and approach that hospice represents fit for almost all the circumstances of my life.

When one of our nurses, Iris Mooreland, was moving out of state, she spoke at the last team meeting she attended about what hospice had meant to her: "I've learned to be comfortable with my uncomfortableness." Maybe that's not perfect grammar, but it struck me as a sharp truth. It's not possible to be totally comfortable with people who are dying and grieving. It will probably always be difficult and complicated.

Hospice has taught us all to rise above our own fears and concerns and focus in on the individual and family and their situation. Later on we can look at our own reactions and questions. Iris also spoke about how important it is to not only suspend our discomfort and fears, but also our judgments. Families have their own ways of doing things and of working things out.

As a hospice nurse, I've thought a lot about the impact on my life of keeping a daily vigil with people who are dying and their families. While hospice work is demanding, there are so many rewards involved in it. So long as the rewards are there to balance out the difficulties, I plan to continue. I don't know where I would find another position that would allow me such opportunities for living my own life so well, and in concert with my own values and beliefs. Hospice has spoiled me for other jobs in nursing.

After eight years, I also realize that I feel like I *belong* with the people at hospice. They are doing the same things that I am, just in different ways, and they respect my contributions. We also talk the same language about some of life's most difficult and mysterious times, and how they influence us as human beings.

Hospice nursing is nursing in its purest form. There's no other kind of nursing I want to do.

—NANCY HOFFMAN

Those whom we support hold us up in life.

—MARIE EBER VON ESCHENBACH

Caring is the greatest thing, caring matters most.

—*Last words of*
FREIDRICH VAN HUGEL

Hospice's Developmental Changes

Hospice care in the United States originally developed out of grassroots efforts in communities where consumers and health care professionals believed there were better and more humane ways of caring for the dying. Some of the early efforts were born out of experiences like Nancy's with her father's death. There was a measure of determination to not only offer people caregiving choices at the end of their life, but also to create the supportive mechanisms to make those caregiving choices possible.

When hospice services developed in the mid-1970s in the United States, there were distinct gaps in the service continuum. While studies at the time showed that the vast majority of people would prefer to die in their home, there were few services to enable that choice. A 1996 Gallup Poll showed that nine out of ten people said they would prefer to be cared for and to die in their home. The poll showed increased understanding of hospice and growing interest in hospice services. So the issues are shifting from the availability of services to awareness and access to hospice services.

There was a belief among early hospice professionals that hospice services and the values and principles they represented would someday become part of mainstream healthcare. Early hospice providers saw themselves as drawing attention to unmet needs as well as serving as constructive agents of change. With the 1982 congressional decision to pay for hospice services under Medicare, hospice care became a distinct, specialized service category. Recent changes in the health care environment have meant increased competition for patients, and new providers, some of them proprietary, beginning to offer hospice services.

In less than thirty years, hospice services have experienced remarkable growth. The people who provide those services have also changed in some ways. Early pioneers of the hospice movement were charismatic individuals with a commitment to improving care of the dying in their local communities. The first hospice professionals were typically volunteers. Reimbursement brought about certification of hospice programs and payment of staff. For many of today's hospice professionals, a job with a hospice program is a pragmatic career opportunity. Because of the payment of staff, hospice workers as a whole are now more diverse and less white, middle class, and female.

In many settings, hospice is still seen as an alternative type of care rather than mainstream medical care. The two elements of hospice care that have been more widely adopted by broader segments of health care providers include approaches to pain and symptom management and the emphasis on home-centered care. Examining the reasons why these principles have been more widely adopted may be less than heartening. Pain and symptom management involves techniques and technologies that can be documented and translated easily into action. The value of a pain-free death is a widely held one, but the gap of actual practice outside of hospice can be great. A recent study of teaching and research hospitals showed that for 50 percent of conscious patients who died in the hospital, family members reported that they experienced moderate to severe pain at least half the time.[2] The technologies for pain and symptom relief exist, but the awareness and understanding of how and when to best utilize them can be alarmingly inadequate.

Hospice was at the beginning of the trend toward home care, which is now widely practiced. Whether or not families have the interest or abilities to provide care, in many health care contexts home care is the only choice offered to them. The motivations that fuel the emphasis upon home care are largely economic rather than those of extending choices or options to consumers. The responsibility of caring for seriously ill persons has shifted from institutions to families. The goal of integrating hospice services and care of the dying into the overall picture of health care services is still a crucial one, a goal that will become increasingly complex and critical in the years to come.

In 1980, the thirteenth year of its operation, St. Christopher's Hospice in Sydenham, England, hosted a conference that explored the development of hospices around the world. Samuel Klagsbrun, M.D., the medical director of Four Winds Hospital in New York, offered three goals that he believed the hospice movement had an obligation to move towards.[3] The first he suggested was to identify and refine the aspects of hospice care that work most successfully, including a focus on the people providing hospice care. Part of this task involves a clearer definition of the unique qualities, including the spiritual dimension, which make up a hospice service.

Secondly, an important present and future goal centers around the application of the hospice approach to a much broader segment of medicine. People suffering from chronic diseases, and people in the "frail elderly," 85–100 age group could benefit from a hospice-like, humanizing approach in the face of diminishing resources and increasing limitations. For most physicians, the shifts in awareness and attitudes represented by the hospice approach have not occurred. Reaching physicians and collaborating with them is essential, not only for hospice services to be made available to families, but also to apply hospice concepts to other appropriate areas of medicine and health care. In a practical sense, physicians need to see that hospice services will benefit them, in addition to benefiting their patients and those patients' families.

A recent federal innovation, the Program of All-inclusive Care for the Elderly (PACE), seeks to prevent unnecessary use of hospital and nursing home care. PACE is a model program, serving persons who are 55 years of age or older in a wide variety of settings. The PACE service-delivery system uses an interdisciplinary team for care management and integrates primary and secondary medical care. Outcomes of PACE programs show a steady census growth, good consumer satisfaction, reduction in the use of institutional care, and cost savings. While the PACE services are available in only a few locations, they are an important step in the incorporation of hospice principles into the broader spectrum of care.

The final goal Klagsbrun suggested was to study how the environment of care that hospice offers impacts the person who is ill and the family members. In addition to the hoped-for improvement in quality-of-life for the person who is dying, hospices need to study the long-term effects on the subsequent life patterns of family members.

These goals are still relevant today. Hospices have refined and clarified their definition of services, and are also seeking to expand the application of the hospice approach through additional services and programs. While hospice has gained wider acceptance, it is still seen as a separate approach from the main structure of care. In spite of many efforts, hospice care has not yet had a major impact on the thinking of most physicians and their treatment of people who are dying. In addition to more research into hospice's successful elements and applications, hospice programs need to extend themselves more into their communities.

Working in Hospice Care

Hospice professionals and volunteers are privy to many of the wide range of learnings that proximity to death and grief offers. That is not to say that people experience personal illness or grief to teach them a particular lesson. Rather, it is a challenge and a responsibility to try to discover and create personal meaning out of our difficult experiences. Discoveries about spirituality, values, and elements of life that are to be explored and treasured are considered to be the life-changing learnings generated by the dying and grieving process. In no way are these learnings to be considered compensatory or worth the distress. In Harold Kushner's book *When Bad Things Happen to Good People*, he concludes with a personal statement acknowledging that in the aftermath of his son Aaron's death, Kushner sees himself as a more compassionate rabbi and a wise teacher who has helped many people. He then unequivocally states that if he had been given a choice in the matter, he would rather have his son back.

While there can be a tendency to romanticize hospice care or make hospice professionals and volunteers into "angels," that idealization may be one more way of distancing from the reality of death and grief. Hospice professionals have chosen to be involved with work that brings them in close contact with issues most people feel an aversion to. There are also some people, both administrators or clinical staff, who work in a hospice principally because it is a good-paying or convenient job. On the other hand, there are a significant number of clinical staff, and the vast majority of volunteers, who are involved with hospice work as a life choice or even a vocation. The reasons for involvement in hospice work are varied. The ones most commonly reported include:

- Care for others in a time of significant need
- Ability to make a positive difference for people who are dying and their families
- Knowledge that the care delivered is better and more compassionate than in past experiences, personal or professional
- Belief in whole-person care
- Interest in interdisciplinary teamwork
- Congruence with personal skills and values
- Commitment to compassion and/or community
- Lower technology, high interaction care
- Challenges of problem-solving and effective symptom-management approaches
- Close involvement with families and dying persons
- Day-to-day reminders about what is important in life
- Encourages a hopeful view of human beings
- Offers opportunities for meaning

Hospice work centers around dramatic and intense life moments. For many hospice professionals and volunteers, it is a way of satisfying personal needs that are important to them. Others see hospice work as an opportunity to serve people in difficult times, thereby maintaining optimism about positive and symbolic human actions. Hospice care is a humane approach that offers specific benefits to people who are dying and their families. In practical and symbolic ways, hospice care offers professionals and volunteers a unique window to human experience that can be both humbling and inspiring.

Professional Coping

Because of the nature of the human situations hospice professionals encounter on a daily basis, significant coping and adaptation skills are required. Bernice Catherine Harper believes that there is a progression of abilities to cope with caring for the dying and bereaved that changes along with one's tenure and increasing comfort. The model Harper developed represents a developmental sequence of emotional and psychological processes involved in working with the dying. Based upon her experience in social work, Harper sees that the growth of understanding, knowledge, strength, and the ability to work through internal and external conflicts expands the personal capacity for caring and helping.[4]

It is widely acknowledged that hospice professionals and volunteers need their own internal and external resources for support, above and beyond those offered by the hospice program. Hospice programs are required by national standards to offer team members access to emotional support to assist them in coping with the losses and changes involved in hospice work.

Care of the dying and bereaved also challenges hospice professionals and volunteers to seek comfort in a dimension beyond the individual and the self. For some, that involves a religious perspective, and for others it centers around an interpersonal focus or a spiritual dimension. For all who work in hospice, there are ongoing attempts to reconcile suffering and death against quality of life and the potential for human caring.

All sorrows can be borne if you put them into a story or tell a story about them.

—ISAK DINESEN

I want by understanding myself, to understand others. I want to be all that I am capable of being . . . This all sounds very strenuous and serious. But now that I have wrestled with it, it's no longer so. I feel happy—deep down. All is well.

—KATHERINE MANSFIELD
1922 journal, last entry

POSTSCRIPT

Because looking at the end of life is difficult, many of us don't contemplate death until its reality is pressing close. For readers who are considering hospice and end-of-life care, we wish you comfort on this powerful journey. Hospice care does not end sorrow or diminish the reality of death. What hospice offers is an approach to ways of being together at the end of life. There is human value and integrity available when we journey with each other through these times.

The stories in this book are true-to-life representations of some of life's most difficult and powerful moments. Personal experiences are always difficult to represent because we can only know a very small part of another person's reality. With deep respect and admiration for the families we have known and worked with, we have tried to show what the end-of-life experience is like for families.

When you love someone, you are able to look past a disease-ridden, emaciated body and see inside the person you know. I will always remember sitting next to Barbara on her bed, with her rose-patterned sheets. She wore a pink turban covering what was left of her thick, curly hair and a T-shirt that my sister Lori and I had bought her that had words about stopping to smell the roses along the way. I was struck by the realization that Barbara was smelling the roses in spite of everything. What I will remember is how sweet the roses were that we enjoyed together, especially in those last months of her life. I see that as a hospice secret: when you look over into the abyss, the important things show themselves to you. That bright-light vision is a secret that can guide the rest of the journey.

I keep the note that Barbara wrote to me before she died in its envelope tucked into the edge of the mirror above my dresser. There is also a rose tucked in a corner that reminds me of my daughter, Ellen, a line from a song that brings my son, Steve, closer, and a picture of my husband, Mike, smiling at me. There are a few other special reminders of people I love, some who are here and some who are gone. I want to remember that love and the time we shared. Those reminders sweeten the beginning and ending of each day when I see them. Perhaps that's what hospice and death have taught me, that we have no guarantees in relationships, but we do witness each other's lives. We live on, representing all the people we have shared life's sweet and sorrowful times with. It's all part of the same story.

This quote became important in the months after my daughter Ellen's death because I felt it somehow mirrored the ways our family tried to live. It gave me comfort and I hope it offers to you a vision of the rewards that are woven into the devotion and commitment that are part of loving someone, living and dying.

—MARCIA LATTANZI-LICHT

Give us the grace and strength to persevere.
Give us courage and gaiety and the quiet mind.
Spare to us our friends and soften to us our
enemies. Give us the strength to encounter
that which is to come, that we may be brave in peril,
constant in tribulation, temperate in wrath and
in all changes of fortune, and down to the gates
of death loyal and loving to one another.

—ROBERT LOUIS STEVENSON

ENDNOTES

Chapter One: Saying Good-bye to Dad

1. Burge, S., and C. R. Figley (1982). *The Social Support Scale*. Unpublished manuscript, Purdue University.
2. Schulz, R. (1978). *The Psychology of Death, Dying and Bereavement*. Reading, MA: Addison-Wesley, pp. 81–82.
3. Frankl, V. E. (1959). *Man's Search for Meaning*. New York: Pocket Books.
4. Ibid.
5. Levy, Michael H. (1996). "Pharmacologic Treatment of Cancer Pain," *NEJM* 335:1124–1132.
6. Portenoy, Russel K. (1996). "Opioid therapy for chronic nonmalignant pain: A review of the critical issues," *Journal of Pain and Symptom Management* 11:203–207.
7. Cassell, Eric J. (1982). "The Nature of Suffering and the Goals of Medicine," *NEJM* 306:639–645.
8. *Standards of a Hospice Program of Care* (1993). Arlington, VA: National Hospice Organization.

Chapter Two: Hospice Care

1. Gallup Poll Survey, 1996. Commissioned by National Hospice Organization.
2. *Journal of the American Medical Association [JAMA]*. November 22/29, 1995.
3. U.S. Department of Health and Human Services, Agency for Health Care Policy and Research. Clinical Practice Guidelines, Number 9. *Management of Cancer Pain*. AHCPR Pub. No. 94-0592. March 1994.
4. *JAMA*. November 22/29, 1995.
5. Kubler-Ross, E. (1969). *On Death and Dying*. New York: Macmillan.
6. *JAMA*. November 22/29, 1995.
7. *Standards of a Hospice Program of Care* (1993). Arlington, VA: National Hospice Organization.
8. Saunders, C. (1988). "The Evolution of the Hospices" in *The History of*

the *Management of Pain: From Early Principles to Present Practice,* R. D. Mann, Ed. Pearl River, NY: Parthenon Publishing Group.

9. Lewis, M. (1989). *Tears and Smiles: The Hospice Handbook.* London: Michael O'Mara Books, Ltd.

10. Ibid, also, W. Phipps (1988) Death Studies 12:91–99.

11. Lewis, *Tears and Smiles.*

12. Kubler-Ross, *On Death and Dying.*

13. Corr, C. (1993), Death Studies 17:69–83.

14. Kubler-Ross, *On Death and Dying.*

15. National Hospice Organization estimates, 1996.

16. Ibid.

17. Federal Register (1993), Vol. 48, No. 243.

18. *Standards of a Hospice Program of Care.*

19. Health Care Financing Administration (1995.). *Hospice Benefits.* HCFA Pub. No. 02154.

20. Lewin-VHI, Inc. (1995). *An Analysis of the Cost Savings of the Medicare Hospice Benefit.* Arlington, VA: National Hospice Organization.

21. Christakis, N. A., and J. J. Escarce, "Survival of Medicare Patients after Enrollment in Hospice Programs." *New England Journal of Medicine* 335:172–8 (1996).

22. Zimmerman, J. (1981). *Hospice, Complete Care for the Terminally Ill.* Baltimore, MD: Urban and Schwarzenberg.

Chapter Three: So Little Time, So Many People

1. Schulz, R. (1978). *The Psychology of Death, Dying and Bereavement.* Reading, MA: Addison-Wesley.

2. Corr, C. A. (1992). *A Task Based Approach to Coping with Dying.* Omega 24:81–94.

3. Saunders, C. M. (1967). *The Management of Terminal Illness.* London: Hospital Medicine.

4. Weisman, A. D. (1979). *Coping with Cancer.* New York: McGraw-Hill.

Chapter Four: My Little One

1. Wilson, D. C., and D. J. English, (1985). "Issues in Hospice Administration," in *Hospice: Development and Administration* (2nd ed.), G. W. Davidson, Ed. Washington, DC: Hemisphere, pp. 83–133.

2. Lattanzi, M. E. (1985). "An Approach to Caring: Caregiver Concerns," in *Hospice Approaches to Pediatric Care,* C. A. Corr and D. M. Corr, Eds. New York: Springer.

3. Lattanzi, M. E. "Hospice Bereavement Services: Creating Networks of Support." *Family and Community Health* 5, No. 3 (November 1982): 54–63.

Chapter Five: The Commitment

1. Weisman, A. D. (1979). *Coping with Cancer*. New York: McGraw-Hill.
2. Harper, B. C. (1977; second edition, 1994). *Death: The Coping Mechanism of the Health Professional*. Greenville, SC: Southeastern University Press.
3. Ferguson, M. (1980). *The Aquarian Conspiracy*. Boston: Houghton Mifflin.
4. Weisman, *Coping with Cancer*, p. 123.
5. Chai, M. (1987). "Older Asians." *Journal of Gerontological Nursing*, (3) 11:11.
6. Merton, T. (1956). *Thoughts in Solitude*. New York: Noonday Press.
7. Steindl-Rast, D. (1996). *A Listening Heart*. New York: Crossroads.
8. Frankl, V. (1959). *Man's Search for Meaning*. New York: Pocket Books.
9. Walker, A. (1989). "Introduction" in *A Rumor of Angels*, G. Perry and J. Perry, Eds. New York: Ballantine, pp. xiii–xv.
10. Yalom I. D. (1980). *Existential Psychotherapy*. New York: Basic Books.
11. Hastings Center Report, November–December, 1995.
12. National Hospice Organization (1996), Position paper on assisted suicide and euthanasia.
13. Hammarskjold, Dag (1964). *Markings*. Translated from the Swedish. New York: Alfred Knopf.

Chapter Six: The Heart Has Reasons

1. Larson, D. G. (1993). *The Helper's Journey*. Champaign, IL: Research Press.
2. Lattanzi, M. E. (1985). "Sustaining Relationships." From the author's Winston Churchill Traveling Fellowship Interviews, Summary report. Boulder, CO.
3. *Standards of a Hospice Program of Care* (1993). Alexandria, VA: National Hospice Organization.
4. Brantner, J. Address to the annual meeting of the National Hospice Organization, Los Angeles, CA, November 1980.
5. Thurman, H. (1947). *Meditations for Apostles of Sensitiveness*. Mills College, CA: Eucalyptus Press.
6. Burrs, F. A. (1995). "The African American Experience: Breaking the Barriers to Hospices." *The Hospice Journal*, 10, no. 2: 15–18.
7. National Hospice Organization's Task Force on Access to Hospice Care by Minorities, (1995). *Caring for Our Own with Respect, Dignity and Love the Hospice Way*. Alexandria, VA: National Hospice Organization.
8. Noggle, B. J. (1995). "Identifying and Meeting Needs of Ethnic Minority Patients." *The Hospice Journal* 10, no. 2: 85–93.
9. Chai, M. (1987). "Older Asians." *Journal of Gerontological Nursing*, (3) 11:11.

10. Saunders, C. (1978). Quoted in S. Stoddard. *The Hospice Movement,* New York: Vintage Books, p. 120.

Chapter Seven: If Wishes Were Horses

1. Parkes, C. M. (1972). *Bereavement: Studies of Grief in Adult Life.* New York: International Universities Press, p. 147.
2. Lasky, N. R., and M. F. Gates, (1994). "Experiences of the Adolescent Caregiver of Cancer Patients." Unpublished raw data. Sigma Theta Tau International.
3. Capossela, C., and S. Warnock, (1995). *Share the Care.* New York: Fireside.
4. Becker, E. (1973). *The Denial of Death.* New York: Free Press.
5. Weisman, A. D. (1972). *On Dying and Denying: A Psychiatric Study of Terminality.* New York: Behavioral Publications.

Chapter Nine: It Doesn't Seem Like Such a Long Time Now

1. Veninga, R. (1985). *A Gift of Hope.* Boston: Little, Brown & Co.
2. Fisher, M. (1995). *I'll Not Go Quietly.* New York: Scribner.
3. National Hospice Organization Statistics (1994). Arlington, VA: National Hospice Organization.
4. Brown, G., and D. Mawn (1996). "Rural Issues" in *Resource Manual for Providing Hospice Care to People Living with AIDS.* Alexandria, VA: National Hospice Organization, pp. 32–39.
5. *Standards of a Hospice Program of Care* (1993). Arlington, VA: National Hospice Organization.
6. Worden, J. W. (1991). *Grief Counseling and Grief Therapy.* New York: Springer.
7. Brenner, P. (1996). "Structuring Response to Losses Due to AIDS" in *Resource Manual for Providing Hospice Care to People Living with AIDS.* Alexandria, VA: National Hospice Organization, pp. 19–26.
8. Fisher, *I'll Not Go Quietly.*

Chapter Ten: Shattered Dreams

1. Connor, S., and M. Lattanzi-Licht (1995). Hospice Trauma Response Survey. Arlington, VA: National Hospice Organization, NewsLine.
2. Ibid.

Chapter Eleven: "I'm a Hospice Nurse"

1. Lattanzi, M. From the author's Winston Churchill Travelling Fellowship, 1984. The information in this story, from this point through the story's end, is a paraphrasing of quotes from the author's Fellowship study.
2. Lynne, J. (1995). "A Controlled Trial to Improve Care for Seriously Ill Hospitalized Patients." *JAMA* 274, no. 20: 1591.

3. Klagsbrun, S. G. (1981). "Hospice—A Developing Role," in *Hospice: The Living Idea*. C. Saunders, D. H. Summers, and N. Teller, Eds. London: Edward Arnold.

4. Harper, B. C. (1977; second edition, 1994). *Death: The Coping Mechanism of the Health Professional*. Greenville, SC: Southeastern University Press.

HOSPICE Q AND A

Q: *Who is eligible for hospice care?*
A: Hospice provides a comprehensive system of care to all terminally ill people and their families regardless of age, gender, nationality, race, creed, sexual orientation, disability, diagnosis, availability of a primary caregiver, or ability to pay. "Terminally ill" is defined by most hospices to suggest that the patient has a prognosis measured in weeks and months. Many insurers, including Medicare, require a prognosis of six months or less for eligibility to a hospice benefit.

Q: *What does the term "palliative" mean?*
A: Hospice defines palliative care as an intensive program of care with the relief of pain and suffering being the treatment goal. When cure is no longer possible, hospice recognizes a peaceful and comfortable death as a valid goal of modern health care. Hospice believes that death is an integral part of the life cycle and that intensive palliative care that focuses on pain relief and comfort is the important goal in the care of dying patients.

Q: *What about chemotherapy, radiation, or other therapy?*
A: The goal of any treatment in hospice is to enhance comfort and improve the quality of the patient's life. No specific therapy is excluded from consideration. The test of treatment lies in the agreement by the patient, the physician, the primary caregiver, and the hospice team that the expected outcome is relief from distressing symptoms, preventing pain, and enhancing the quality of life. The

decision to intervene with an active treatment is based on the treatment's ability to meet the stated goals rather than its effect on the underlying disease.

Q: *Can everyone access hospice care?*
A: Almost. While hospice care only began in the United States in 1974, the majority of states have full coverage of hospice services available to residents. There remain a few geographic areas of the nation that do not have service, but as programs continue to expand, those areas are decreasing. To find out if you have hospice services in your area, call the Hospice HelpLine at (800) 658-8898.

Q: *When should a decision about entering a hospice program be made and who should make it?*
A: At any time during a life-limiting illness, it's appropriate to discuss all of a patient's care options, including hospice. By law, the decision belongs to the patient or the patient's surrogate.

Q: *Should I wait for our physician to raise the possibility of hospice, or should I raise it first?*
A: The patient and family should feel free to discuss hospice care at any time with their physician, other health care professionals, clergy, or friends.

Q: *What if our physician doesn't know about hospice?*
A: Most physicians are familiar with hospice, even if they have not worked directly with a hospice program. If your physician needs additional information, contact the National Hospice Organization for references in your area or national hospice physician groups as identified in the resources section of this book.

Q: *Can a hospice patient who shows signs of recovery be returned to regular medical treatment?*
A: Yes. If the patient's condition improves and the disease seems to be in remission, patients can be discharged from hospice and return to active therapy. If a discharged

patient should later need to return to hospice care, Medicare and most private insurance will allow additional benefit coverage for this purpose.

Q: *What does a hospice admission process involve?*
A: One of the first things hospice will do is contact the patient's physician to make sure he or she agrees that hospice care is appropriate. (Hospices have medical staff available to help patients who have no physician.) The patient will also be asked to sign consent and insurance forms; these are similar to forms patients sign when they enter a hospital. It also outlines the services available.

Q: *Is there any special equipment or changes I have to make in my home before hospice care begins?*
A: Your hospice provider will work with you to assess your needs and recommend and help make arrangements for any necessary equipment. Often the need for equipment is minimal at first and increases as the disease progresses. In general, hospice will assist in any way it can to make home care as convenient and safe as possible.

Q: *How many family members or friends does it take to care for a patient at home?*
A: There is no set number. One of the first things a hospice team will do is to prepare an individualized care plan that will, among other things, address the amount of caregiving needed in your situation. Hospice staff visit regularly and are always accessible to answer medical questions and provide support.

Q: *Must someone be with the patient at all times?*
A: In the early weeks of care, it's usually not necessary for someone to be with the patient all the time. Later, however, since one of the most common fears of patients is the fear of dying alone, it is generally recommended that someone be with the patient continuously. While family and friends must be relied on to give most of the care,

hospices can provide volunteers to assist with errands and to provide a break and time away for major caregivers.

Q: *How difficult is caring for a dying loved one at home?*

A: It's never easy and sometimes can be quite hard. At the end of a long, progressive illness, nights especially can be very long, lonely, and scary. So, hospices have staff available around the clock to consult with the family and make night visits if the need arises.

Q: *Is caring for the patient at home the only place hospice care can be delivered?*

A: No. Although 90 percent of hospice patient time is spent in a personal residence, some patients live in a nursing home, assisted living facility, hospice care centers, or other group quarters. In addition, some hospice programs provide day-care programs.

Q: *How does hospice manage pain?*

A: Hospice believes that emotional and spiritual pain are just as real and in need of attention as physical pain, so it addresses each. Pain, as much as possible, is addressed prior to need, thus preventing it rather than responding to it. Hospice physicians, nurses, and pharmacists are up to date on the latest medications, devices, and options for pain- and symptom-relief. In addition, physical and occupational therapists assist patients to be as mobile and self-sufficient as possible, and are often joined by specialists schooled in music therapy, art therapy, massage, and diet counseling.

Q: *Is hospice affiliated with any religious organizations?*

A: Hospice is not based on any specific religious organization. While some churches and religious organizations have started hospices, sometimes in connection with other health care programs, these hospices serve a broad community and do not require patients to adhere to any particular set of beliefs.

Q: *Is hospice care covered by insurance?*

A: Insurance coverage for hospice care is widely available. Hospice will assist families in finding out whether the patient is eligible for coverage. Coverage is provided by Medicare nationwide, by Medicaid in thirty-eight states, and by most private health insurance policies. Medicare covers all services and supplies related to the hospice patient's terminal illness. In some hospices, the patient may be required to pay a 5 percent or $5 copayment on medication and respite care. Most hospices will provide for anyone who cannot pay using money raised from the community or from memorial or foundation gifts.

Q: *Does hospice provide any support to the family after the patient dies?*

A: Hospice provides continuing contact and support for family and friends for at least a year following the death of a loved one. Most hospices also provide specialized bereavement programs and more and more are becoming the major community resource for bereavement services.

Q: *What are the qualifications of hospice staff to meet the variety of needs of patients and their families?*

A: All team members meet appropriate degree and/or licensure standards of the state and of federal program requirements for Medicare (if the program is Medicare-certified). In addition, the majority of hospice staff members across the nation are experienced in caring for dying people and their families, are familiar with working with people in their own personal residences, and, more than anything, are caring and understanding people.

Q: *How can hospice help with specific diseases and decision-making?*

A: Often, hospice staff can help patients and families answer questions about end-of-life care planning and decision-making. Families caring for a family member with Alzheimer's disease often need help with determining when a patient should or could be admitted to hospice care. Families in this situation are often very tired, and they want to be sure they are asking the right questions and have access to comprehensive information. Patients with end-stage renal disease often desire counseling about options related to stopping dialysis, and about the next steps to take after that decision might be made.

Q: *Are all hospice programs the same?*

A: The majority of hospice programs across the nation provide very similar core services, and if they are certified by Medicare, you can be assured that these core services are all provided. Many programs, however, provide additional services that are reflective of the needs of the community, the size of the hospice program, the community resources that are available, or the partnerships that have been created with other organizations in the community to support the needs of the dying and their families.

Q: *I know we have more than one hospice in our community; how do we select the right one to meet our needs?*

A: In most cases, an individual patient/family will not need to search out a hospice program to serve them. Many communities now have several hospice programs to serve the needs of the terminally ill, and many are associated with local hospitals or have referral arrangements with physician practices and managed care organizations. Your physician, hospital discharge planner, clergyperson, or social worker can refer you to a hospice program that serves your area. You can also call the NHO-sponsored Hospice HelpLine (800/658-8898). When choosing a hospice program, care should be taken to determine that the hospice is certified to provide services under the Medicare Hospice Benefit. Even if the patient does not qualify for Medicare, such certification is an indication of the comprehensive nature of the services that the hospice provides. If the state requires licensure, the hospice should be able to provide evidence that it complies with

all state licensing requirements. Many hospices are
accredited by the Joint Commission on Accreditation of
Healthcare Organizations (JCAHO), the Community
Health Accreditation Program, Inc. (CHAPS), and other
accrediting organizations. Ask for evidence of such
accreditation.

Q: *How might one "advance plan" for hospice care?*

A: Learning about hospice care is the most effective way to
advance plan for when hospice care may be needed by an
individual or family member. The more you know about
the hospice in your community, the better equipped you
are to make appropriate decisions for end-of-life care for
yourself, family members, friends, and colleagues. A terminal diagnosis or the advancement to a terminal stage of
a chronic illness often creates an environment surrounded
by turmoil. Having advance information about hospice
care will assist in effective decision-making during this
time. While learning about hospice care in your community, you may also find ways to become involved in supporting care for others with a terminal illness and their
families even though you don't have a direct need for services at a specific time.

Q: *How long is hospice care usually needed?*

A: It depends on many factors. Some patients only receive
hospice care for a few days, as they are admitted when
their disease has progressed to a point where they are
actively dying, and thus may not receive the full benefit of
care that is available to the patient and the family. Others
receive hospice care for a number of months prior to
death. Often, patients will have a period where they do
better after being admitted to a hospice program, as they
respond to hospice's focus on palliation rather than
endure curative therapies. Patients also vary in the
amount of time they are in stages of active dying; with
some the process takes only a few hours and with others,
several days.

Q: *What will family members see in their loved ones as death approaches and is there anything family members can do to make their loved one more comfortable?*

A: As death approaches, various signs or symptoms may appear: 1) increased sleep; 2) change in breathing; 3) decreased circulation in the extremities; 4) withdrawal or detachment from others; 5) congestion in the lungs or throat; 6) restlessness; 7) confusion; 8) incontinence; 9) visionlike experiences; 10) decreased intake of fluid and foods; 11) decreased urine output; and 12) lowered body temperature. The chart below provides responses that may make your loved one more comfortable during this time. Dying people usually experience these signs at different times and in varying degrees.

SIGNS OF APPROACHING DEATH*

Sign	Comfort Action
Coolness	Cover loosely but not with an electric blanket
Somnolence/increased sleepiness	A normal reaction. Sit with the patient.
Confusion	Speak softly, clearly, and truthfully
Incontinence	Catheter, chux, or adult diapers
Congestion in lungs or throat	Position head to the side, clear mouth/airway. Medication or suction may be used if necessary, may raise head of bed.
Restlessness	Light massage, quiet voice, soothing music. Protect from injury.
Withdrawal or detachment from others	Give space, encourage interpersonal communication to extent comfortable to person.
Visionlike experiences	Do not discount. Ask for details. Try to understand symbolic meanings and reassure them they are safe and not alone.

Sign	Comfort Action
Decreased intake of fluid and foods	Give supplements as tolerated. Pay attention to presentation of food and fluides. Maintain good mouth care.
Decreased urine output	Observe intake and output. Urine will become darker, consider a foley catheter. Usually a sign that death is nearing.
Changes in breathing	Irregular breathing, periods of not breathing, panting, and wet respirations. Elevate the head, turn patient on side. Hold hand. Speak gently.

*Chart adapted from *Hospice Practice, Pitfalls and Promise,* by S. R. Connor (Taylor & Francis: Washington, D.C., 1998).

CONSUMER INFORMATION AND RESOURCES

National Hospice Organization

THE NATIONAL HOSPICE ORGANIZATION (NHO) was created to promote the hospice concept of care, to ensure the quality of that care, and to help make it available for every terminally ill American who needed it. These goals have been pursued by providing leadership, information, training, and advocacy for the many hospice programs that care for dying persons and their families in communities across the country.

NHO was founded in 1978 as a nonprofit, public-benefit, charitable organization advocating for the needs of terminally ill persons in America. NHO is the oldest and largest independent national nonprofit membership organization devoted exclusively to hospice care in the U.S. NHO's current membership includes 2,100 hospice programs, 48 state hospice organizations (plus the District of Columbia), and more than 4,000 individual professionals.

NHO's organizational vision is to profoundly enhance the end of life for people dying in America by ensuring access to quality hospice care. NHO's mission is to educate about and advocate for the fundamental *philosophy* and *principles* of hospice care to meet the unique needs of each terminally ill person and his or her family.

NHO's organizational goals are to:

- Serve as the nationally-recognized voice of hospice
- Act as the national steward and guardian for the definition, values, application, integrity, influence, and accessibility of hospice care
- Influence health programs and public policies relative to hospice care and the needs of the terminally ill and their families
- Provide educational programs, publications, technical assistance, and other services consistent with the philosophy and principles of hospice care
- Increase public awareness and understanding of the philosophy and principles of hospice care
- Contribute significantly to the theoretical and practical knowledge of hospice, end-of-life care and concerns, and aspects of grief and loss
- Promote hospice care to the general public
- Maintain a comprehensive and viable professional organization capable of achieving our mission

Standards of a Hospice Program of Care

The National Hospice Organization has established the following *Standards of Hospice Program of Care* to lead quality of care within hospice programs across the nation:

ACCESS TO CARE . Hospice offers palliative care to all terminally ill people and their families regardless of age, gender, nationality, race, creed, sexual orientation, disability, diagnosis, availability of a primary caregiver, or ability to pay.

PATIENT/FAMILY AS THE UNIT OF CARE   Hospices care for the dying person and the family.

HOSPICE INTERDISCIPLINARY TEAM   A highly qualified, specially trained team of hospice professionals and volunteers work together to meet the physical, psychological, social, and spiritual needs of patients/families facing terminal illness and bereavement.

INTERDISCIPLINARY TEAM PLAN OF CARE The hospice interdisciplinary team collaborates continuously with the person who is dying, family members, and with the patient's attending physician to develop and maintain an individualized, coordinated plan of care.

SCOPE OF HOSPICE SERVICES Hospice offers a safe, coordinated program of palliative and supportive care, in a variety of appropriate settings, from the time of admission through bereavement, with the focus on keeping terminally ill patients in their own homes as long as possible.

COORDINATION AND CONTINUITY OF CARE Hospice care is available twenty-four hours a day, seven days a week, and services continue without interruption if the patient care setting changes.

UTILIZATION REVIEW Hospice is accountable for the appropriate allocation and utilization of its resources in order to provide optimal care consistent with patient/family needs.

HOSPICE SERVICES RECORD Hospice maintains a comprehensive and accurate record of services provided in all care settings for each patient/family.

GOVERNING BODY Hospice has an organized governing body that has complete and ultimate responsibility for the organization.

MANAGEMENT AND ADMINISTRATION The hospice governing body entrusts the hospice administrator(s) with overall management responsibility for operating the hospice, including planning, organizing, staffing, and evaluating the organization and its services.

QUALITY ASSESSMENT AND IMPROVEMENT   Hospice is committed to continuous assessment and improvement of the quality and efficiency of its services.

Medicare Hospice Certification—"Conditions of Participation"

The Health Care Financing Administration (HCFA) defines hospice "conditions of participation" for eligibility as a Medicare Certified Hospice. Certification of a hospice program is necessary to receive Medicare reimbursement for hospice services. Categories of conditions that broadly define the structure of hospice services include:

General Provisions and Administration

- Governing body
- Professional management
- Medical director
- Plan of care
- Continuation of data
- Informed consent
- In-service training
- Quality assurance
- Interdisciplinary group
- Volunteers
- Licensure
- Central clinical records

Core Services

- Nursing services
- Physician services
- Medical social services
- Counseling services

Other Services

- Physical therapy, occupational therapy, and speech-language therapy
- Home health aide and homemaker services
- Medical supplies
- Short-term inpatient care
- Hospices that provide inpatient care directly

The Conditions of Participation also list qualifications of hospice personnel and contain definitions of terms used in the document. These categories of services are translated into specific practice elements that are carefully reviewed by state certifiers on an annual basis.

Current Hospice Statistics*

- Approximately one out of every seven deaths (14.8 percent) in America from all causes (not just terminal illness) were cared for by a hospice program.
- Fifty-two percent of hospice patients are male.
- Forty-eight percent of hospice patients are female.
- Of the male patients, 71 percent were 65 or older; 23 percent between 39 and 64; 8 percent were 18 to 34; and 1 percent were 17 or younger.
- Of the female patients, 74 percent were 65 or older, 21 percent between 45 and 64, 6 percent were 18 to 44; and 1 percent were 17 or younger.
- Sixty percent of hospice patients had cancer.
- Six percent of hospice patients had heart-related diagnoses.
- Four percent of hospice patients had AIDS.
- Two percent had renal (kidney) diagnoses.
- Two percent had Alzheimer's disease.

*Based on the 1992 and 1995 NHO Hospice Census.

- Twenty-six percent were diagnosed with other non-cancer diseases or conditions.
- Hospices care for about one out of every two cancer and AIDS deaths in America.
- Patients, on average, spend approximately fifty-seven days being cared for by a hospice program.
- Eighty-four percent of hospice patients were white, 9 percent were African-American, 4 percent were Hispanic, 1 percent Asian, and 2 percent were identified as "other."
- Sixty-three percent of patients were married, 35 percent were single, and 2 percent had unknown marital status.
- Fifty-five percent of hospice patients lived with their spouse, 20 percent lived with children, 10 percent lived with a significant other, 10 percent lived alone, and 5 percent lived with parents.
- Seventy-seven percent of hospice patients died in their own personal residence; 20 percent died in facilities, including inpatient hospice facilities; 3 percent died in other settings.
- Fifty-five percent of hospice patients/families use the volunteer services that are offered to them.
- Fifty-nine percent of volunteer hours were provided in direct support of patients.

NHO Resource and Contact Information

National Hospice Organization
1901 North Moore Street, Suite 901
Arlington, VA 22209
(703) 243-5900
The Nation's only advocacy organization dedicated to advancing the fundamental principles and philosophies of hospice care.

Hospice HelpLine

(800) 658-8898

General information about hospice, the Medicare Hospice Benefit, and referrals to hospice programs providing care in the United States.

National Hospice Organization Internet HomePage

http://www.nho.org

The NHO HomePage provides comprehensive information on end-of-life care. This database also includes referral information including referral contact phone number for hospice programs serving your area. Other features include general information about hospice care, Medicare Hospice Benefit, educational information, and information on activities of the National Hospice Foundation. From this site, you can link to other sites related to care for people at the end of life.

National Council of Hospice Professionals

1901 North Moore Street, Suite 901

Arlington, VA 22209

(703) 243-5900

The only national organization dedicated to enhancing the integrity of the hospice interdisciplinary team by advancing the development of hospice professionals.

National Hospice Foundation

1901 North Moore Street, Suite 901

Arlington, VA 22209

(703) 243-5900

The national foundation dedicated to expanding America's vision for end-of-life care. Program areas include public outreach, professional education, and research.

State Hospice Organizations

Each state also has a hospice organization that will provide information and resources for patients and families; please contact the Hospice HelpLine at (800) 338-8619 to access information on the state hospice organization in your state.

RESOURCE GROUPS

AIDS National Interfaith Network
110 Maryland Avenue, NE, Suite 504
Washington, DC 20002
(202) 546-0807

Alzheimer's Disease and Related Dementia Association of America
919 North Michigan Avenue
Chicago, IL 60611
(312) 335-5790

American Academy of Hospice and Palliative Medicine
P.O. Box 14288
Gainesville, FL 32604
(352) 377-8900

American Association of Retired Persons—Widowed Persons Service
601 E Street, NW
Washington, DC 20049
(800) 424-3410

American Cancer Society
1519 Clifton Road, NE
Atlanta, GA 30329
(404) 320-3333

American Heart Association
727 Greenville Avenue
Dallas, TX 75231
(214) 373-6300 / (800) 242-8721

Amyotropic Lateral Sclerosis (ALS) Association
21021 Ventura Boulevard, Suite 321
Woodland Hills, CA 91364
(800) 782-4747

Australian Association for Palliative Care, The
P.O Box 1200, North Fitzroy
Victoria, 3068, Australia
61-3-486-2666

Canadian Palliative Care Association
43 Bruyer Street, Suite 112
Ottowa, Ontario, K195C8, Canada
(613)-560-1483

**Cancer Information Service—National Cancer
Institute/National Institutes of Health**
9000 Rockville Pike, Building 31, 10A24
Bethesda, MD 20892
(800) 4-CANCER

Centers for Disease Control—National AIDS Clearinghouse
P.O. Box 6003
Rockville, MD 20850
(800) 458-5231

Children's Hospice International
2202 Mt. Vernon Avenue, Suite 3C
Alexandria, VA 22301
(703) 684-0330

Choice in Dying
200 Varick Street
New York, NY 10014
(212) 366-5540

The Compassionate Friends
P.O. Box 3696
Oakbrook, IL 60522
(708) 990-0010

Eldercare Locator—National Association of Area Agencies on Aging
1112 16th Street, NW, Suite 100
Washington, DC 20036
(800) 677-1116

European Association for Palliative Care
National Cancer Institute
Milan, via Venezian 1, 20133
Milan, Italy
39-2-2390-243-534

The Family Caregiver Alliance
425 Bush Street, Suite 500
San Francisco, CA 94108
(415) 434-3388

Hospice and Palliative Care Nurses Association
5512 Northumberland Street
Pittsburgh, PA 15217
(412) 687-3231

Hospice Association of America
519 C Street, NE
Washington, DC 20002
(202) 546-4759

Hospice Education Institute
P.O. Box 713
Essex, CT 06426
(800) 331-1620

Hospice Foundation of America
777 17th Street, Suite 401
Miami Beach, FL 33139
(305) 538-9272

Leukemia Society of America
600 Third Avenue
New York, NY 10016
(800) 955-4LSA

National Alliance of Breast Cancer Organizations
9 East 37th Street, 10th Floor
New York, NY 10016
(212) 889-0606

National Alliance for Caregiving
7201 Wisconsin Avenue, Suite 620
Bethesda, MD 10814
(301) 718-8144

National Association of People with AIDS
1413 K Street, NW
Washington, DC 20005
(202) 898-0414

National Chronic Pain Outreach Association
7979 Old Georgetown Road, Suite 100
Bethesda, MD 20814
(301) 652-4948

National Consumers League
815 15th Street, NW, Suite 928-N
Washington, DC 20005
(202) 639-8140

National Council on Aging
409 3rd Street, SW, Suite 200
Washington, DC 20024
(800) 424-9046

National Family Caregivers Association
9621 East Bexhill Drive
Kensington, MD 20895
(800) 896-3650

National Funeral Directors Association
11121 West Oklahoma Avenue
Milwaukee, WI 53227
(800) 228-6332

National Hospice Organization
1901 North Moore Street, Suite 901
Arlington, VA 22209
(703) 243-5900
http://www.nho.org

National Organization of Victim Assistance
1757 Park Road, NW
Washington, DC 20010
(202) 232-6682

Rosalynn Carter Institute
Georgia Southwestern College
800 Wheatley Street
Americas, GA 31709
(912) 928-1234

Social Security Administration
Baltimore, MD 21235
(800) 772-1213

ADDITIONAL READING

American Cancer Society. *Caregiving for the Patient with Cancer—at Home.*

Arnold, Johann Christophe. *I Tell You a Mystery: Life, Death, Eternity.* Farmington, PA: Plough Publishing House, 1996.

Beresford, Larry. *The Hospice Handbook.* Boston: Little Brown, 1993.

Bernardin, J. *The Gift of Peace.* Chicago: Loyala Press, 1997.

Birkendahl, Nonie. *Older & Wiser: A Workbook for Coping with Aging.* Oakland, CA: New Harbinger, 1991.

Brooks, T. *Signs of Life.* New York: Times Books, 1997.

Byock, Ira. *Dying Well.* New York: Riverhead Books, 1997.

Callahan, Maggie, and Patricia Kelley. *Final Gifts.* New York: Simon & Schuster, 1992.

Capossela, Cappy, and Sheila Warnock. *Share the Care.* New York: Simon & Schuster, 1995.

Carter, Rosalynn, with Susan Golant. *Helping Yourself Help Others: A Book for Caregivers.* New York: Random House, 1994.

Connor, S. R. *Hospice Practice Pitfalls.* Washington, DC: Taylor & Francis, 1997.

Das, Ram and Paul Gorman. *How Can I Help?* New York: Alfred A. Knopf, 1985.

Davidson, Glen W. *Living with Dying: A Guide for Relatives and Friends.* Minneapolis: Augsburg Fortress, 1975.

Davies, B., J. C. Reimer, P. Brown, and N. Martens. *Fading Away: The Experience of Transition in Families with Terminal Illness.* Amityville, NY: Baywood, 1996.

Donnely, Katherine Fair. *Recovering from the Loss of a Sibling.* New York: Dodd, Mead, & Co., 1988.

Edison, Ted, Ed. *The AIDS Caregiver's Handbook.* New York: St. Martin's Press, 1986.

Felder, Leonard. *When a Loved One Is Ill: How to Take Better Care of Your Loved One, Your Family, and Yourself.* New York: Penguin, 1991.

Fisher, Mary. *I'll Not Go Quietly.* New York: Scribner, 1995.

Fumia, Molly. *Safe Passage.* Berkeley, CA: Conari Press, 1992.

Gasta, L. L., with C. Post. *A Graceful Exit: Life and Death on Your Own Terms.* New York: Plenum Press, 1996.

Harper, Bernice Cathering. *Death: The Coping Mechanism of the Health Professional.* Greenville, SC: Southeastern University Press, 2nd ed., 1994.

Harwell, Amy. *Ready to Live—Prepared to Die.* Wheaton, IL: Shaw Publishers, 1995.

Heiss, Gayle. *Finding the Way Home: A Compassionate Approach to Illness.* Fort Bragg, CA: QED Press, 1997.

de Hennezel, M. *Intimate Death.* New York: Alfred A. Knopf, Inc., 1995.

Herman, Judith Lewis. *Trauma and Recovery.* New York: Basic Books, 1992.

Horne, Jo. *When Caring Becomes Caring for . . . A Survival Guide for Family Caregivers.* Minneapolis: CompCare Publishers, 1991.

Jaffe, C., and C. Ehrlich. *All Kinds of Love: Experiencing Hospice.* Amityville, NY: Baywood, 1997.

Knapp, Ronald J. *Beyond Endurance: When a Child Dies.* New York: Schocken Books, 1986.

Kramer, Kay and Herbert. *Conversations at Midnight.* New York: Avon Books, 1993.

Krementz, Jill. *How It Feels When a Parent Dies.* New York: Knopf, 1992.

Kushner, Harold. *When Bad Things Happen to Good People.* New York: Avon, 1984.

Larson, Dale G. *The Helper's Journey.* Champaign, IL: Research Press, 1993.

Lederman, Ellen. *Making Life More Livable.* New York: Simon & Schuster, 1994.

Levine, Steven. *Healing into Life & Death.* New York: Anchor, 1987.

Lewis, C. S. *A Grief Observed.* New York: Bantam Books, 1976.

Madden, Edward F. *Carpe Diem: Enjoying Every Day with Terminal Illness.* Boston: Jones & Bartlett, 1993.

Management of Cancer Pain. U.S. Department of Health and Human Services, Public Health Service, Agency for Health Care Policy and Research, Rockville, MD: 1994.

Maurer, Linda K. *Standing Beside You.* Boulder, CO: Johnson Printing, 1996.

Nuland, Sherwin B. *How We Die.* New York: Random House, 1993.

Nungessor, Lon G. *Axioms for Survivors: How to Live Until You Say Goodbye.* San Bernadino, CA: Borgo Press, 1990.

Peck, M. S. *Denial of the Soul.* New York: Harmony Books, 1997.

Ray, M. Catherine. *I'm Here to Help.* Mound, MN: Hospice Handouts, 1992.

Ray, M. C. *I'm with You Now.* New York: Bantam Books, 1997.

Rosof, Barbara D. *The Worst Loss.* New York: Henry Holt & Co., 1995.

Saunders, C., and R. Kastenbaum. *Hospice Care on the International Scene.* New York: Springer Publishing Co. Inc., 1997.

Saunders, Catherine M. *Surviving Grief.* New York: John Wiley & Sons, 1992.

Sharp, J. *Living Our Dying.* New York: Hyperion, 1996.

Shneidman, Edwin. *Voices of Death.* New York: Kodansha, 1995.

Stoddard, Sandol. *The Hospice Movement: A Better Way of Caring for the Dying.* New York: Stein & Day, 1978.

Veninga, Robert. *A Gift of Hope: How We Survive Our Tragedies.* New York: Ballantine, 1985.

Viorst, Judith. *Necessary Losses.* New York: Simon & Schuster, 1986.

Watson, Jeffrey. *The Courage to Care—Helping Aging, Grieving, and Dying.* Grand Rapids, MI: Baker Book House, 1992.

Whitman, Juliet. *Breast Cancer Journal.* Golden, CO: Fulcrum, 1993.

INDEX

Printed in the United States
31573LVS00005B/9